MEASUREMENT OF JOINT MOTION:

A GUIDE TO

GONIOMETRY

MEASUREMENT OF JOINT MOTION:

A GUIDE TO

GONIOMETRY

CYNTHIA CLAIR NORKIN, Ed.D., R.P.T.

ASSOCIATE PROFESSOR AND DIRECTOR, SCHOOL OF PHYSICAL THERAPY
OHIO UNIVERSITY, COLLEGE OF HEALTH AND HUMAN SERVICES
CONVOCATION CENTER
OHIO UNIVERSITY
ATHENS, OHIO

D. JOYCE WHITE, M.S., R.P.T.

CLINICAL ASSISTANT PROFESSOR OF PHYSICAL THERAPY
SARGENT COLLEGE OF ALLIED HEALTH PROFESSIONS
BOSTON UNIVERSITY
BOSTON, MASSACHUSETTS

PHOTOGRAPHS BY LUCIA GROCHOWSKA LITTLEFIELD

ILLUSTRATIONS BY JENNIFER DANIELL
AND MEREDITH TAYLOR STELLING

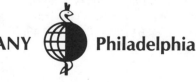

F. A. DAVIS COMPANY Philadelphia

Printed in the United States of America

Last digit indicates print number: 10 9 8

Library of Congress Cataloging in Publication Data

Norkin, Cynthia C.
  Measurement of joint motion.

  Bibliography: p.
  Includes index.
  1. Joints—Range of motion—Measurement. I. White, D. Joyce. II. Title. [DNLM: 1. Joints—physiology. 2. Movement. WE 300 N841m]
RD734.N67 1985   612'.75   84-14985
ISBN 0-8036-6578-4

DEDICATION

To Carolyn, Alexandra, and Jonathan
Without their support and encouragement this book would not have been possible.

PREFACE

The measurement of joint motion is an important component of a comprehensive physical examination of the extremities and spine, which enables health professionals to accurately assess dysfunction and rehabilitative progress. Considerable time is spent in many educational programs teaching goniometric evaluation. The lack of an appropriate text on goniometry has forced instructors to expend a great deal of effort not only in preparing their own teaching material, but also in demonstrating testing positions, stabilization techniques and goniometer alignments. Students often have difficulty remembering specific aspects of the instructor's demonstrations and may not have adequate resources available for study purposes.

Measurement of Joint Motion: A Guide to Goniometry evolved from teaching materials on goniometry originally prepared in 1974 for physical therapy students at Boston University. During the following years of teaching experience in goniometry, the need for a comprehensive, well-illustrated goniometry text that went beyond a compendium with line sketches became increasingly evident. In the early 1980s, the decision was made to undertake a major revision and expansion of the original teaching materials for the purpose of publication. The book that resulted is appropriate for use in a wide variety of educational programs for health professionals. Although designed as an instructional text, the book is also useful as a reference guide in the clinical setting.

The book presents goniometry in a logical, clear manner. Chapter 1 defines anatomic motions and discusses elements of active and passive range of motion. The inclusion of end-feels introduces the learner to current concepts in orthopedic manual therapy and encourages the learner to consider joint structure while he or she is measuring joint motion. A discussion of reliability and validity of measurement helps to convey the importance of using standardized goniometric evaluation procedures.

Chapter 2 takes the learner through a step-by-step procedure to master the technique of goniometric evaluation. Included are exercises that help to develop necessary psychomotor skills and that demonstrate direct application of theoretical concepts.

Chapters 3, 4, and 5 present detailed information on goniometric evaluation of the upper and lower extremities, spine, and temporomandibular joint. Each of these last three chapters is divided into sections on testing position, stabilization, physiologic end-feel, and goniometer alignment for each joint; this format reinforces a consistent approach to evaluation. The extensive use of photographs and captions should eliminate the need for repeated demonstrations by the instructor. The photographs provide the learner with a permanent reference for visualizing the procedures. The opened book lies flat on a table and therefore can be easily used in a laboratory and in a clinical setting.

We hope this book will make the teaching and learning of goniometry easier and improve the standardization and thus the reliability of this evaluative tool.

CCN

DJW

ACKNOWLEDGMENTS

We wish to express our appreciation to the following people for their invaluable assistance in the preparation of this book.

To photographer Lucia Littlefield we owe a special debt of gratitude. Her patience, good humor, and friendship helped to carry us through the many picture-taking sessions that extended over a two-year period. Lucia's good-natured willingness to pursue excellence combined with her talents is responsible for the high quality photographs that comprise a major portion of the book.

To Jennifer Daniell, a recent Boston University graduate in physical therapy, who, through her artistic talents and knowledge of the subject matter, produced the line drawings in Figures 1-2 through 1-6 and Figures 2-10 and 2-11, we are also very indebted.

To Meredith Taylor Stelling, a recent Harvard University graduate, who gave freely of her talent, time, and effort to produce the line drawings that appear in Figure 1-1 and Figures 2-3 through 2-5, we are most grateful.

To Claudia Van Bibber, who was a subject for some of the photographs, we extend our thanks.

CONTENTS

INTRODUCTION TO GONIOMETRY

OBJECTIVES

Upon completion of this chapter the reader will be able to:

1. **Define the following terms:**
   goniometry
   planes and axes
   range of motion
   end-feel
   reliability
   validity

2. **Identify the appropriate planes and axes for each of the following motions: flexion-extension, abduction-adduction, and rotation.**

3. **Compare:**
   active and passive ranges of motion
   reliability and validity
   intratester and intertester reliability
   soft, firm, and hard normal end-feels

This text is designed to serve as a guide to learning the technique of human joint measurement called **goniometry.** This technique is used by many different evaluators of human function such as physical and occupational therapists, athletic trainers, physical educators, biomedical engineers, orthotists, and physicians. Goniometric measurements provide the examiner with kinematic data about the joints of the body.

>   Example: Goniometric data may be used by an examiner as a partial basis for:
>   - developing treatment goals
>   - evaluating progress or lack of progress toward goals
>   - modifying treatment
>   - motivating the subject
>   - researching the effectiveness of specific therapeutic techniques or regimens, for example, exercises, medications, and surgical procedures
>   - fabricating orthoses and adaptive equipment

In addition to goniometry, a comprehensive joint evaluation should include a history of injury or symptoms, pain assessment, observation for normal alignment, contour and skin color, and palpation and special tests to assess associated soft tissue structures. Information derived from the preceding tests used in conjunction with goniometric data should provide a comprehensive picture of a joint.

DEFINITIONS

GONIOMETRY

The term goniometry is derived from two Greek words, *gonia,* meaning angle, and *metron,* meaning measure. Goniometric measurements may be used to determine both a particular joint position and the total amount of motion available at a joint. These measurements are obtained by placing the parts of the measuring instrument along the proximal and distal bones adjacent to the joint under consideration.

>   Example: The elbow joint is evaluated by placing the parts of the measuring instrument on the humerus (proximal component) and the forearm (distal component) and measuring either a specific joint position or the total arc of motion (Fig. 1-1).

PLANES AND AXES

Motions at a joint are described as taking place in one of the three cardinal planes of the body (sagittal, frontal, and transverse) around three corresponding axes (coronal, anterior-posterior, and longitudinal). The three planes lie at right angles to one another, while the three axes lie at right angles both to one another and to their corresponding planes.

The sagittal plane extends from the anterior to the posterior aspect of the body and the median sagittal plane di-

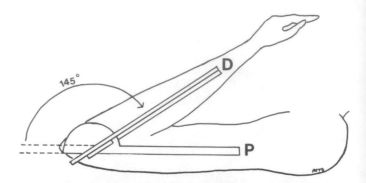

FIGURE 1-1. This figure shows the upper left extremity of a subject in the supine position. The humerus (proximal component) is designated by the letter (P). The forearm (distal component) is designated by the letter (D). The parts of the measuring instrument have been placed along the proximal and distal components and centered over the axis of the elbow joint. When the distal component has been moved toward the proximal component (elbow flexion), a measurement of the arc of motion can be obtained.

vides the body into right and left halves. The motions of flexion and extension occur in the sagittal plane.

The axis around which the motions of flexion and extension occur may be conceived of as a line that is perpendicular to the sagittal plane and which extends from one side

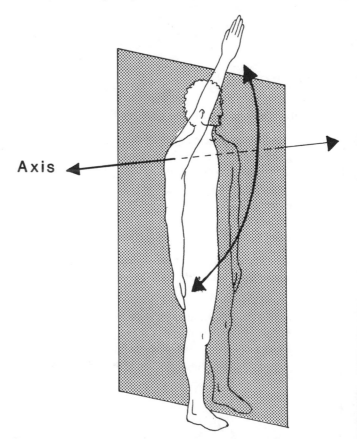

FIGURE 1-2. The shaded areas in the illustration indicate the sagittal plane. This plane extends from the anterior aspect of the body to the posterior aspect. Motions in this plane, such as flexion and extension of the upper and lower extremities, take place around a coronal axis.

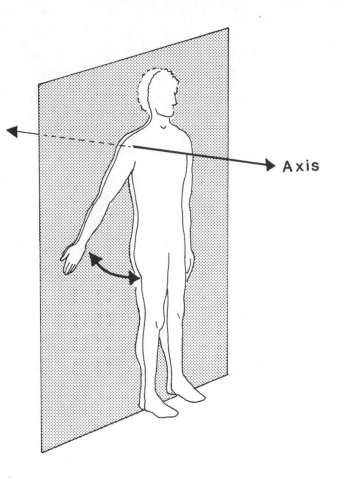

FIGURE 1-3. The frontal plane, which is indicated by the shaded area, extends from one side of the body to the other. Motions in this plane, such as abduction and adduction of the upper or lower extremities, take place around an anterior-posterior axis.

of the body to the other. This axis is called a coronal axis, and all motions in the sagittal plane take place around a coronal axis.

Example: Flexion and extension occur in the sagittal plane around a coronal axis (Fig. 1-2).

The frontal plane, which extends from one side of the body to the other, is the plane in which the coronal axis lies. The terms frontal and coronal are synonymous, but in this manual the term frontal is used to describe the plane, while the term coronal is used to describe the axis. The frontal plane lies at right angles to the sagittal plane and divides the body into front and back halves. The motions that occur in the frontal plane are abduction and adduction.

The axis around which the motions of abduction and adduction take place is an anterior-posterior axis. This axis lies at right angles to the frontal plane and extends from the anterior to the posterior aspect of the body. Therefore the anterior-posterior axis lies in the sagittal plane.

Example: Abduction and adduction are motions that occur in the frontal plane around an anterior-posterior axis (Fig. 1-3).

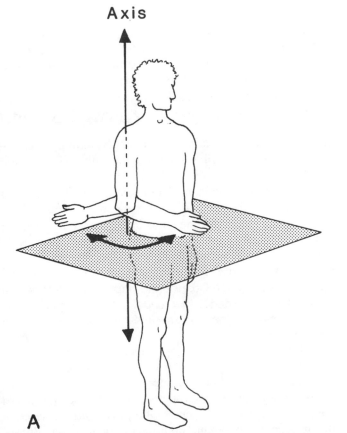

A

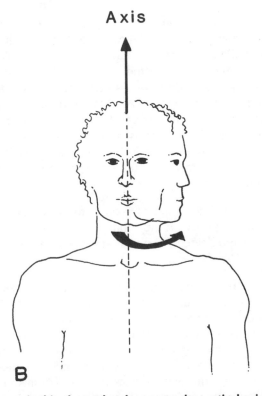

B

FIGURE 1-4. The horizontal plane is indicated by the shaded area (A). Movements in this plane take place around a vertical axis. These motions include rotations of the head (B), shoulder, and hip, as well as pronation and supination of the forearm (A).

The transverse plane is horizontal and divides the body into upper and lower portions. The motion of rotation occurs in the transverse plane around a longitudinal axis, which lies at right angles to the transverse plane and extends vertically in a craniocaudal direction.

Example: Medial and lateral rotation occur in the transverse plane around a longitudinal axis (Fig. 1-4A and B).

The motions described in the examples are pure motions because they occur in a single plane around a single axis. Combination motions such as circumduction (flexion-extension-abduction-adduction) are possible at many joints, but because of the limitations imposed by the uniaxial design of the measuring instrument, only pure motions are measured in goniometry.

The amount as well as the type of motion that is available at a joint varies according to the structure of the joint. Some joints, such as the interphalangeal joints of the digits, permit motion in only one plane around a single axis: flexion and extension in the sagittal plane around a coronal axis. Other joints, such as the glenohumeral joint, permit motion in three planes around three axes: flexion and extension in the sagittal plane around a coronal axis; abduction and adduction in the frontal plane around an anterior-posterior axis; and medial and lateral rotation in the transverse plane around a longitudinal axis.

The planes and axes for each joint and joint motion to be measured are presented for the reader in Chapters 3 to 6.

RANGE OF MOTION

The amount of motion that is available at a specific joint is called the range of motion (ROM). The starting position for measuring all ROMs, except rotations, is the anatomic position. In this body position the upper and lower extremity joints are at zero degrees for flexion-extension and abduction-adduction (Fig. 1-5A). A body position in which the extremity joints are halfway between medial (internal) and lateral (external) rotation is zero degrees for the ROM in rotation (Fig. 1-5B). When a ROM begins at zero degrees it proceeds in an arc toward 180 degrees[1] as shown in the following example.

Example: The range of motion for shoulder flexion, which begins with the shoulder in the anatomic position (zero degrees) and ends at full flexion, is expressed as 0–180 degrees.

In the preceding example, the portion of the extension ROM from full shoulder flexion back to the zero starting position does not need to be measured, because this ROM represents the same arc of motion as was measured in flexion. However, the portion of the extension ROM that is available beyond the zero starting position must be measured (Fig. 1-6). The term extension, as it is used in this manual, refers to both the motion that is a return from full flexion to the zero starting position and the motion that normally oc-

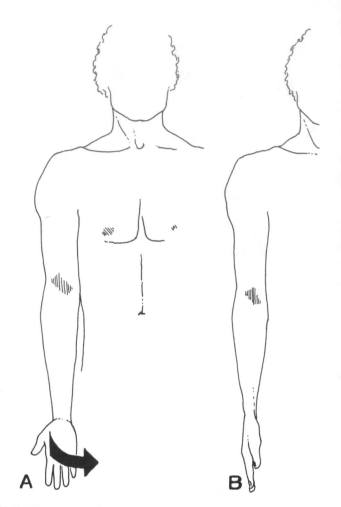

FIGURE 1-5. *A,* In the anatomic position the forearm is supinated so that the palms of the hands face anteriorly. *B,* When the forearm is in a neutral position (with respect to rotation), the palm of the hand faces the side of the body.

appendix A p 138
avg. range of motion

curs beyond the zero starting position. The term hyperextension is used to describe a greater than normal extension ROM.

The ROM varies considerably among individuals and may be affected by age and sex among other factors.[1-7] Average ranges of motion for the joints of the body may be found in the handbook of the American Academy of Orthopaedic Surgeons[8] and a variety of other texts.[9-16] However, the average ranges of motion found in many of these texts should serve only as a guide because the populations from which the averages were derived are undefined or the specific testing positions and type of instruments that were used are not identified.

Because standardized age- and sex-related norms for average ROMs for all of the joints in this manual have not been established, information on average ROMs for specific joints is not included in Chapters 3 to 6. The reader should refer to Appendix A or to one of the texts or articles listed in the references to obtain information on average ROMs. However, an examiner should not allow knowledge of normal values to bias test results.

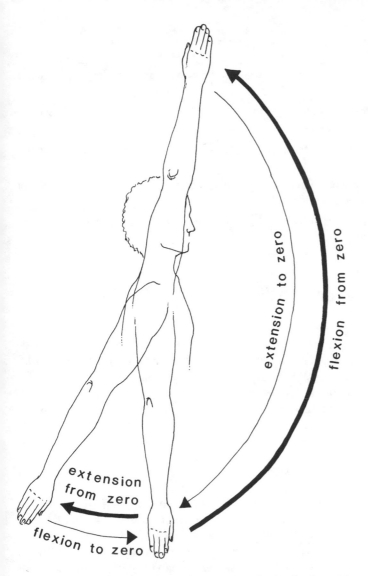

extension to zero

flexion from zero

extension from zero

flexion to zero

FIGURE 1-6. Shoulder flexion and extension. Flexion begins with the shoulder in the anatomic position and the forearm in the neutral position (PALM OF HAND FACES THE BODY). The ROM in flexion extends from the zero position through an arc of 180 degrees. The long, dark arrow shows the ROM in flexion that is measured in goniometry. The short, dark arrow shows the ROM in extension that is measured in goniometry.

The ROM, in addition to being affected by age, sex, and other factors, is affected by the type of motion being performed (passive or active).

A PASSIVE RANGE OF MOTION is the amount of motion attained by an examiner without any assistance from a subject during the performance of a joint motion. Normally, the passive ROM is slightly greater than the active ROM, because each joint has a small amount of available motion (joint play motion) that is not under voluntary control. The additional passive ROM that is available at the end of the normal active ROM helps to protect joint structures, because it allows the joint to give and absorb extrinsic forces.

Testing the passive ROM provides the examiner with information about the integrity of the articular surfaces and

the extensibility of the joint capsule, associated ligaments, and muscles. Therefore, the passive ROM always should be tested in goniometry. The passive ROM should be tested prior to performing a manual muscle test, because the grading of muscle tests is based upon completion of a joint ROM. An examiner needs to know the extent of the ROM before initiating a manual muscle test. *→ muscle strength*

The ACTIVE RANGE OF MOTION refers to the amount of joint motion that is attained by a subject during the performance of unassisted voluntary joint motion. Testing the active ROM provides the examiner with additional information regarding a joint, including muscle strength and movement coordination. Assessment of the active ROM is important for providing information about a subject's functional ability, but the active ROM usually is not tested in goniometry. *★ willingness to do motion*

Example: An examiner may find that a subject with a muscle paralysis has a full passive ROM but no active ROM at the same joint. In this instance, nothing is wrong with the joint surfaces or the extensibility of the joint capsule, ligaments, or muscles. The lack of muscle strength is preventing active motion at the joint.

In cases of disability such as muscle paralysis the passive and active ROMs may vary considerably. Comparisons between the passive and active ROMs provide information about the amount of motion permitted by the joint structure (passive ROM) relative to the person's ability to produce motion at a joint (active ROM). If one wishes to compare a passive ROM with an active ROM, the testing position, stabilization, goniometer alignment, and type of goniometer should be the same for each measurement.

END-FEEL *- what you feel at end. what's limiting motion?*

The extent of the passive ROM is determined by the unique structure of the joint being tested. Some joints are structured so that the joint capsules limit the end of the ROM in a particular direction, while other joints are structured so that ligaments limit the end of a particular ROM. Other limitations to motion include contact of joint surfaces, passive or reflexive muscle tension, and soft tissue approximation.

Each specific structure that serves to limit a range of motion has a characteristic feel to it, which may be detected by the examiner who is performing the passive ROM. This feeling, which is experienced by an examiner as a resistance to further motion at the end of a passive ROM, is called the end-feel. The examiner's ability to distinguish among different types of end-feels requires practice and sensitivity. Determination of the end-feel of a joint must be carried out slowly and carefully in order to detect the particular character of the end-feel and to distinguish among the various physiologic (normal) and pathologic (abnormal) end-feels. Cyriax,[17] Kaltenborn,[18] and Paris[19] have described a variety of physiologic and pathologic end-feels.[20] Tables 1-1 and 1-2 have

 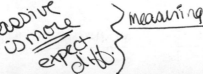

TABLE 1-1. Physiologic (Normal) End-Feels

END-FEEL	STRUCTURE	EXAMPLE
Soft	Soft tissue approximation	Knee flexion (contact between soft tissue of posterior leg and posterior thigh)
Firm	Muscular stretch	Hip flexion with the knee straight (passive elastic tension of hamstring muscles)
	Capsular stretch	Extension of metacarpophalangeal joints of fingers (tension in the anterior capsule)
	Ligamentous stretch	Forearm supination (tension in the palmar radioulnar ligament of the inferior radioulnar joint, interosseous membrane, oblique cord)
Hard	Bone contacting bone	Elbow extension (contact between olecranon process of the ulna and the olecranon fossa of the humerus)

been adapted from the works of these authors. Readers should practice trying to distinguish among the end-feels so that they will be able to determine when the end of a ROM occurs and what type of end-feel exists (see Chapter 2, exercise I).

In Chapters 3 to 6 we have described what we believe to be the physiologic end-feel and the structures that limit the ROM for each joint. Because of the paucity of specific literature in this area, these descriptions are based upon our experience in evaluating joint motion and on information obtained from established anatomy[21,22] and biomechanics texts.[11-13,23-25] In some parts of the body, such as the hand, there is considerable controversy among experts concerning the structures that limit the ROM. Also, normal individual variations in body structure may cause instances in which the end-feel will differ from our description. In any case, we believe it is important to begin to define the end-feels and limiting structures for each joint and motion, and we welcome communication in this area from our readers.

RELIABILITY

Joint measurements that are used either as a basis for treatment planning or for research purposes must be RELIABLE and VALID. RELIABILITY of joint measurement refers to the amount of agreement between successive measurements of the same joint: the higher the amount of agreement between measurements, the higher the reliability. The two types of reliability that are important in goniometry are intratester reliability and intertester reliability.

INTRATESTER RELIABILITY refers to the amount of agreement between measurements of the same joint by the same tester. The reliability of goniometric measurements has been investigated and intratester reliability is higher than intertester reliability.[2,3,26,27] Both types of reliability have been found to be higher for upper extremity joint measurements at the shoulder, elbow, and wrist than for lower extremity measurements at the hip, knee, and ankle.[3]

TABLE 1-2. Pathologic (Abnormal) End-Feels

END-FEEL		EXAMPLES
Soft	Occurs sooner or later in the ROM than is usual; or in a joint that normally has a firm or hard end-feel. Feels boggy.	Soft tissue edema Synovitis
Firm	Occurs sooner or later in the ROM than is usual; or in a joint that normally has a soft or hard end-feel.	Increased muscular tonus Capsular, muscular, ligamentous shortening
Hard	Occurs sooner or later in the ROM than is usual; or in a joint that normally has a soft or firm end-feel. A bony grating or bony block is felt.	Chondromalacia Osteoarthritis Loose bodies in joint Myositis ossificans Fracture
Empty	No real end-feel because end of ROM is never reached because of pain. No resistance is felt except for patient's protective muscle splinting or muscle spasm.	Acute joint inflammation Bursitis Abscess Fracture Psychogenic in origin

muscle guarding- don't want do do it.

INTERTESTER RELIABILITY refers to the amount of agreement between measurements of the same joint by different testers: the higher the amount of agreement (less variability) between measurements, the higher the reliability of the measurement.

VALIDITY — *as close to reality as we can make it.*

VALIDITY of joint measurement may be determined by answering the following question: How closely does an obtained joint measurement represent the actual angle or total available range of motion? (A valid joint measurement is one that truly represents either the actual joint angle or the total range of motion, as determined within the limits of the testing instrument.) If two successive joint measurements are in agreement, they are considered reliable. However, they are not considered valid unless they truly represent the actual joint angle or ROM. Sometimes joint measurements may be reliable but not valid (within the limits of the testing instrument).

The reliability and validity of goniometric measurement may be enhanced by the use of specific procedures. For example, two examiners using the same procedures to measure the same ROM are more likely to obtain the same or similar values than if each examiner had used different procedures to measure the same joint ROM. This manual is designed to help the reader learn the procedures necessary for producing reliable and valid joint measurements.

[ex.] — measure on real person the measure on x-ray.

TECHNIQUES AND PROCEDURES

OBJECTIVES

Upon completion of this chapter the reader will be able to:

1. Explain the importance of the following:
   recommended testing positions
   stabilization
   clinical estimates
   recording starting and ending positions

2. Describe:
   the parts of the goniometer

3. List:
   the six-step explanation sequence
   the twelve-step testing sequence
   the ten items included in recording

4. Perform a goniometric evaluation of the elbow joint including:
   a clear explantion of the procedure
   positioning of a subject in the recommended testing position
   adequate stabilization of the proximal joint component
   a correct determination of the end of the range of motion
   a correct identification of the end-feel
   palpation of the correct bony landmarks
   accurate alignment of the goniometer
   correct reading of the goniometer and recording of the measurement
5. Perform intratester and intertester reliability tests.

Competency in goniometry requires that the reader acquire the following knowledge and develop the following skills.

KNOWLEDGE

The reader must have knowledge of the following for each joint and motion:

1. Recommended testing positions
2. Alternative positioning
3. Stabilizations required
4. Joint structure and function
5. Normal end-feels
6. Anatomic bony landmarks
7. Instrument alignment

SKILLS

The reader must be able to perform the following for each joint and motion:

1. Position and stabilize correctly
2. Move a part through the appropriate range of motion
3. Determine the end of the range of motion (end-feel)
4. Palpate the appropriate bony landmarks
5. Align the measuring instrument with landmarks
6. Read the measuring instrument
7. Record measurements correctly

TECHNIQUES

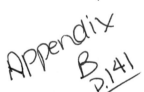
Appendix B P. 141

POSITIONING

Positioning is an important part of goniometry, because it is used to place the joints in a zero starting position and to help stabilize joint components. Positioning affects the amount of tension that is present in soft tissue structures surrounding a joint (capsule, ligaments, and tendons). Adopting a position in which one or more of these soft tissue structures are or will become taut results in a more limited ROM than using a position in which the same structures are or will become lax.

If examiners use the same position during successive measurements of a joint ROM, the relative amounts of tension present in the soft tissue structures should be the same as in previous measurements. Therefore, a comparison of ROMs taken in the same position should yield reliable results.[27] When different testing positions are used for successive measurements of a joint ROM, no basis for comparison exists. As can be seen in the following example, the use of different testing positions significantly alters the ROM obtained for ulnar and radial deviation of the wrist.

> Example: A position in which the shoulder is abducted and the elbow is flexed yields significantly greater ranges of radial and ulnar deviation than a test position in which the shoulder is adducted and the elbow flexed.[28]

Recommended testing positions refer to the positions of the body that we are recommending for obtaining goniometric measurements. As yet, standardized goniometric testing positions have not been established, and testing positions vary considerably among authors. The series of recommended testing positions that are presented in this text are designed to:

1. place a joint at zero degrees
2. provide stabilization for the proximal joint component
3. permit a complete range of motion

If a recommended testing position cannot be attained because of restrictions imposed by the environment or limitations of the subject, the examiner must use his or her creativity to decide how to obtain a particular joint measurement. The alternative testing position that is created must serve the same three functions as the recommended testing position. Also, the examiner must describe the position precisely so that the same position can be used for all subsequent measurements.

Recommended testing positions involve a variety of different positions. When an examiner intends to test a number of joints and motions during one testing session, the goniometric examination must be planned to avoid moving the subject unneccessarily. For example, if the subject is prone, all possible measurements in this position should be taken before moving the subject into another position. The chart in Appendix B that lists joint measurements by body position has been designed to help the examiner plan a goniometric examination.

STABILIZATION

The recommended testing position helps to stabilize the subject's body and proximal joint component so that a motion can be isolated to the joint under consideration. Isolating the motion helps to insure that a true measurement of the ROM results rather than a measurement of combined motions that occur at a series of joints. However, the stabilization provided by the recommended position is often insufficient and must be supplemented by manual stabilization provided by the examiner.

> Example: Measurement of medial (internal) rotation of the hip joint is performed with the subject in a recommended sitting position. The pelvis (proximal component) is stabilized by the body weight, but the subject's trunk and pelvis may move during hip rotation (Fig. 2-1A).
>
> Additional stabilization may be provided by the examiner and the subject. The examiner may provide manual stabilization for the pelvis by exerting a downward pressure on the iliac crest on the side being tested (Fig. 2-1B). The subject may be instructed to shift weight over the hip being tested in order to keep the pelvis stabilized.

The amount of manual stabilization applied by an examiner must be sufficient to keep the proximal joint compo-

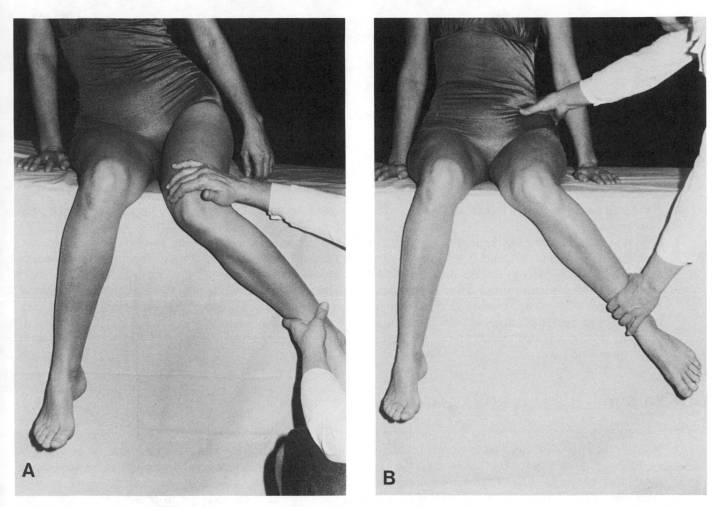

FIGURE 2-1. *A,* This photograph illustrates the consequences of inadequate stabilization. The examiner has failed to stabilize the subject's pelvis and trunk; therefore, a lateral tilt of the pelvis and lateral flexion of the trunk accompanies the motion of hip internal rotation. The range of internal rotation appears greater than it actually is because of the added motion from the pelvis and trunk. *B,* This photograph illustrates the use of proper stabilization. The examiner is using her right hand to stabilize the pelvis (keep the pelvis from raising off the table) during the passive range of motion. The subject is instructed to assist in stabilizing the pelvis by placing her weight on the left side. The subject is asked to keep her trunk straight by placing both hands on the table.

nent fixed during movement of the distal joint component. If both the distal and proximal joint components are allowed to move during joint testing, the end of the range of motion cannot be determined. Learning how to stabilize requires practice, because the examiner must stabilize with one hand while simultaneously moving the distal joint component with the other hand. The techniques of stabilizing the proximal joint component and of determining the end of a range of motion (end-feel) are basic to goniometry and must be mastered prior to learning how to use the goniometer. Exercise 1 is designed to help the reader learn how to stabilize and how to determine the end of the range of motion (end-feel).

EXERCISE 1. DETERMINING THE END OF THE ROM AND END-FEEL

This exercise is designed to help the reader determine the end of the range of motion and to differentiate among the three physiologic (normal) end-feels: soft, firm, and hard.

ELBOW FLEXION—SOFT END-FEEL

1. Select a partner.
2. Position your partner supine with the arm placed close to the side of the body. A pad is placed under the distal end of the humerus to allow full elbow extension. The forearm is placed in full supination with the palm of the hand facing the ceiling. Move the subject's forearm toward the humerus (flex elbow).

3. With one hand, stabilize the distal end of the humerus (proximal joint component) to prevent flexion of the shoulder.
4. With the other hand, slowly move the forearm through the full passive range of elbow flexion until you feel resistance limiting the motion.
5. Gently push against the resistance until no further flexion can be achieved. Carefully note the quality of the resistance. This soft end-feel is caused by compression of the muscle bulk of the anterior forearm with that of the anterior upper arm.
6. Compare this soft end-feel with the soft end-feel found in knee flexion (see knee flexion in Chapter 4).

ANKLE DORSIFLEXION—FIRM END-FEEL

1. Select a partner.
2. Place your partner sitting so that the lower leg is over the edge of the supporting surface and the knee is flexed at least 30 degrees.
3. With one hand stabilize the distal end of the tibia and fibula to prevent knee extension and hip motions.
4. With the other hand on the plantar surface of the metatarsals, slowly move the foot through the full passive range of ankle dorsiflexion until you feel resistance limiting the motion.
5. Push against the resistance until no further dorsiflexion can be achieved. Carefully note the quality of the resistance. This firm end-feel is caused by tension in the Achilles tendon, the posterior portion of the deltoid ligament, posterior talofibular ligament, the calcaneofibular ligament, and the posterior joint capsule.
6. Compare this firm end-feel with the firm end-feel found in metacarpophalangeal extension of the fingers (see Chapter 3).

ELBOW EXTENSION—HARD END-FEEL

1. Select a partner.
2. Position your partner supine with the arm placed close to the side of the body. A pad is placed under the distal end of the humerus to allow full elbow extension. The forearm is placed in full supination with the palm of the hand facing the ceiling. Move the subject's forearm toward the humerus (flex elbow).
3. With one hand, stabilize the distal end of the humerus (proximal joint component) to prevent extension of the shoulder.
4. With the other hand, slowly move the forearm through the full passive range of elbow extension until you feel resistance limiting the motion.
5. Gently push against the resistance until no further extension can be attained. Carefully note the quality of the resistance. When the end-feel is hard it has no give to it. This hard end-feel is caused by contact between the olecranon process of the ulna and the olecranon fossa of the humerus.
6. Compare this hard end-feel with the hard end-feel usually found in radial deviation of the wrist (see radial deviation in Chapter 3).

USING THE GONIOMETER

The instrument most commonly employed for obtaining goniometric measurements is called a GONIOMETER. Many different types of commercially produced, manually operated goniometers are available. These manually operated instruments may be purchased from most surgical and medical supply companies. Electrogoniometers,[29,30,31] which are more sophisticated instruments than manually operated goniometers, are used primarily in research to obtain dynamic joint measurements and therefore will not be discussed in this text.

Manually operated goniometers may be constructed of metal or plastic. These instruments are produced in many sizes and shapes but adhere to the same basic design (Fig. 2-2). Typically, the design includes a BODY and two thin extensions called ARMS—a STATIONARY ARM and a MOVING ARM (Fig. 2-3).

The BODY of the goniometer resembles a protractor and may form a full or half circle (Fig. 2-4). Measuring scales are located on one or on both sides of the body. Sometimes two scales are located on each body surface. The scales on a full-circle instrument extend either from 0 to 180 degrees and 180 to 0 degrees or from 0 to 360 degrees and from 360 to 0 degrees. The scales on a half-circle instrument extend from 0 to 180 degrees and from 180 to 0 degrees. The intervals on the scales may vary from 1 to 10 degrees.

Traditionally, the ARMS of the goniometer are designated as MOVING or STATIONARY according to their method of attachment to the body. The STATIONARY ARM is a structural part of the body and cannot be moved independently of the body. The MOVING ARM is attached to the fulcrum in the center of the body by a screwlike device which permits the arm to move freely on the body. In some instruments the screw may be tightened to hold the moving arm in a certain position or loosened to allow free move-

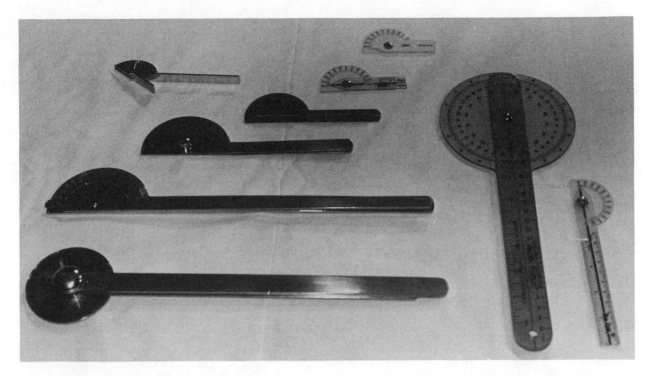

FIGURE 2-2. Metal and plastic manually operated goniometers are available in different sizes and shapes. The goniometer on the far right side of the photograph is a half-circle plastic goniometer. The goniometer at the far left top of the photograph is a metal goniometer designed for measuring the range of motion of the small joints of the fingers and toes. The two small plastic goniometers at the top of the photograph also may be used to measure the range of motion of the fingers and toes. The two metal goniometers pictured at the bottom of the photograph, as well as the large full-circle plastic goniometer, are used to measure motion at large joints such as the knee and hip.

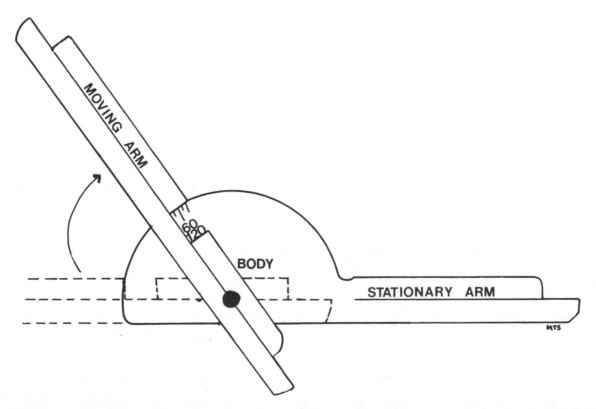

FIGURE 2-3. The body of the goniometer in the illustration forms a half-circle. The stationary arm is an integral part of the body in this particular type of goniometer and cannot be moved independently. The moving arm is attached to the body by either a screw or rivet; therefore, the moving arm can be shifted without an accompanying movement of the body. The moving arm in the illustration has a cut-out portion that is sometimes referred to as a window. The window permits one to read the scale on the body of the instrument.

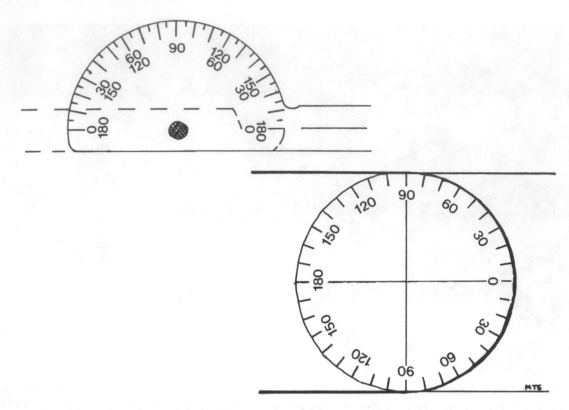

FIGURE 2-4. The body of the goniometer may form either a half circle *(top)* or a full circle *(bottom)*.

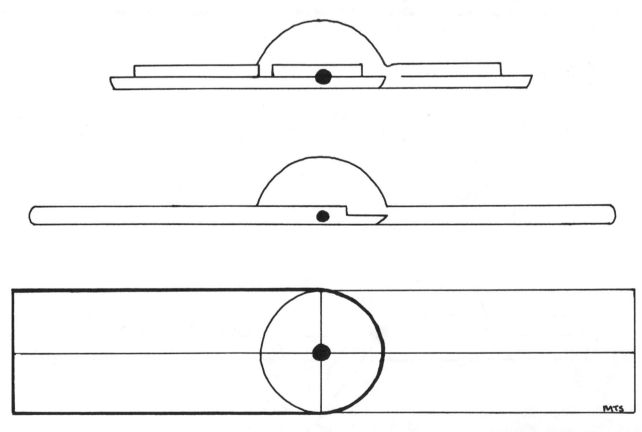

FIGURE 2-5. The half-circle goniometer pictured at the top of the illustration possesses a number of features that facilitate reading of measurements. The moving arm has a black line that extends the length of the arm and cut-out portions at either end and in the middle of the moving arm. The half-circle goniometer in the middle of the illustration has a cut-out portion at the end of the moving arm. The full-circle plastic goniometer at the bottom of the illustration has a black line that extends along the middle of both the moving and stationary arms.

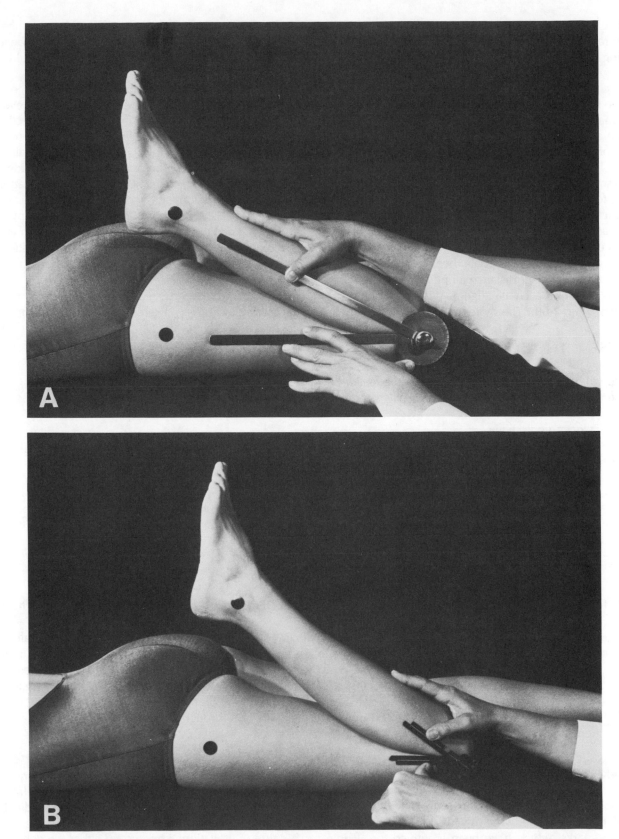

FIGURE 2-6. *A,* The selection of a goniometer of the appropriate size is an important consideration in joint measurement. A full-circle goniometer with long arms has been selected to measure the range of motion of knee flexion. The arms of the goniometer extend along the distal and proximal components of the joint to within a few inches of the bony landmarks (black dots) that are used to align the arms. The proximity of the ends of the arms to the landmark makes alignment easy and insures that the arms are aligned accurately. *B,* The small half-circle metal goniometer being employed to measure the range of motion of knee flexion represents an inappropriate choice on the part of the examiner. The landmarks are located so far from the ends of the arms of the goniometer that accurate alignment of the arms is impossible.

ment. The moving arm may have one or more of the following features: a pointed proximal end, a black or white line extending the length of the arm, or a cut-out portion (window) (Fig. 2-5). These features help the user to read the scales.

The length of the arms varies among instruments from approximately 3 to 16 inches. These variations in length represent an attempt on the part of the manufacturers to adapt the size of the instrument to the size of the joints.

Example: A goniometer with 16-inch arms is appropriate for measuring motion at the knee joint, because the arms are long enough to permit alignment with the greater trochanter of the femur and the lateral malleolus of the tibia (Fig. 2-6A). A goniometer with short arms would be inappropriate, because the arms do not extend a sufficient distance along either the femur or tibia to permit accurate alignment with the bony landmarks (Fig. 2-6B). The same long arms would be inap-

propriate for measurement of the metacarpophalangeal joints of the hand, because the arms would be too long to align with the phalangeal and metacarpal bones.

Estimates of a joint position or range of motion can be obtained by simple observation. These estimates, even when produced by a skilled clinician, yield only subjective information, in contrast to goniometric measurements, which yield objective information. However, clinical estimates are useful in the learning process. Such estimates made prior to goniometric measurements help to reduce errors attributable to reading the goniometer incorrectly. Goniometric measurements of a ROM can be compared with the approximate ROM obtained through observation. If the goniometric measurement is not in the same quadrant as the estimate, the examiner is alerted to the possibility that the wrong scale is being read.

After the reader has read and studied this section on the measuring instrument, Exercise 2 should be completed.

EXERCISE 2. THE GONIOMETER

The following activities are designed to help the reader become familiar with the goniometer.
Equipment: Full-circle and half-circle goniometers made of plastic and metal.
Activities:
1. Select a goniometer.
2. Identify the type of goniometer selected by noting the shape of the body (full-circle and half-circle).
3. Differentiate between the moving and stationary arms of the goniometer. (Remember the stationary arm is an integral part of the body.)
4. Observe the moving arm to see if it has a cut-out portion.
5. Find the line in the middle of the moving arm and follow it to a number on the scale.
6. Study the face on the body and answer the following questions:
   Is the scale located on one or both sides?
   Is it possible to read the scale through the face of the goniometer?
   What intervals are used?
   Does the face contain one or two scales?
7. Hold the goniometer in both hands. Position the arms so that they form a continuous straight line. When the arms are in this position, the goniometer is at 0 degrees.
8. Keep the stationary arm fixed in place and shift the moving arm while watching the numbers on the scale, either at the tip of the moving arm or in the cut-out portion. Shift the moving arm from 0 to 45, 90, 150, and 180 degrees.
9. Keep the stationary arm fixed and shift the moving arm from 0 degrees through an estimated 45-degree arc of motion. Compare the estimate with the actual arc of motion by reading the scale on the goniometer. Try to estimate other arcs of motion and compare the estimates with the actual arc of motion.
10. Keep the moving arm fixed in place and move the stationary arm through different arcs of motion.
11. Repeat numbers 2 through 10 using different goniometers.

ALIGNMENT

GONIOMETER ALIGNMENT refers to the alignment of the arms of the goniometer with ANATOMIC LANDMARKS. These landmarks, which have been identified for all joint measurements, should be exposed so that they may be identified easily (Fig. 2-7). Use of these landmarks in conjunction with recommended testing positions should increase the accuracy and reliability of goniometric measurements. The landmarks and the test positions must be learned and closely adhered to as far as possible.

The STATIONARY ARM is often aligned parallel to the longitudinal axis of the proximal portion of the joint, and the MOVING ARM is aligned parallel to the longitudinal axis of the distal portion of the joint (Fig. 2-8). In some situations, because of limitations imposed by either the goniometer or the patient (Fig. 2-9A), it may be necessary to reverse the alignment of the two arms so that the moving arm is aligned with the proximal part, while the stationary arm is aligned with the distal portion (Fig. 2-9B). Therefore, we have decided to use the term PROXIMAL ARM to refer to the arm of the goniometer that is aligned with the proximal portion of

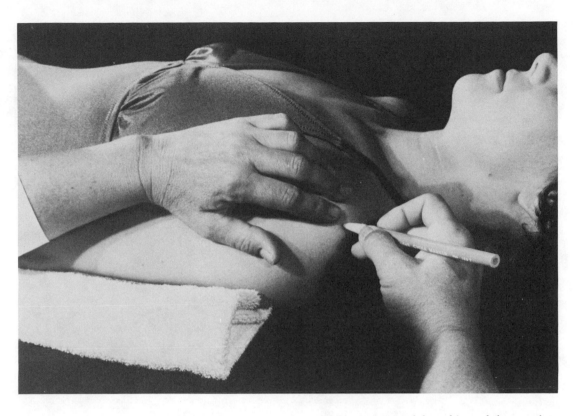

FIGURE 2-7. The examiner in the photograph is using a grease pencil to mark the location of the subject's left acromion process. Notice that the examiner is using the second and third digits of her left hand to palpate the bony landmark.

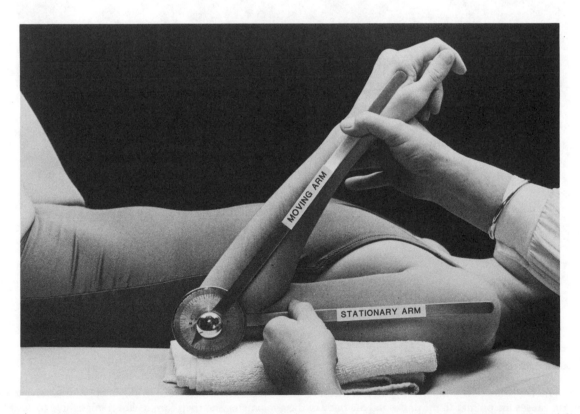

FIGURE 2-8. When a full-circle goniometer is used to measure the range of motion of elbow flexion, the stationary arm of the goniometer is aligned parallel to the longitudinal axis of the proximal part (subject's left humerus), and the moving arm is aligned parallel to the longitudinal axis of the distal part (subject's left forearm).

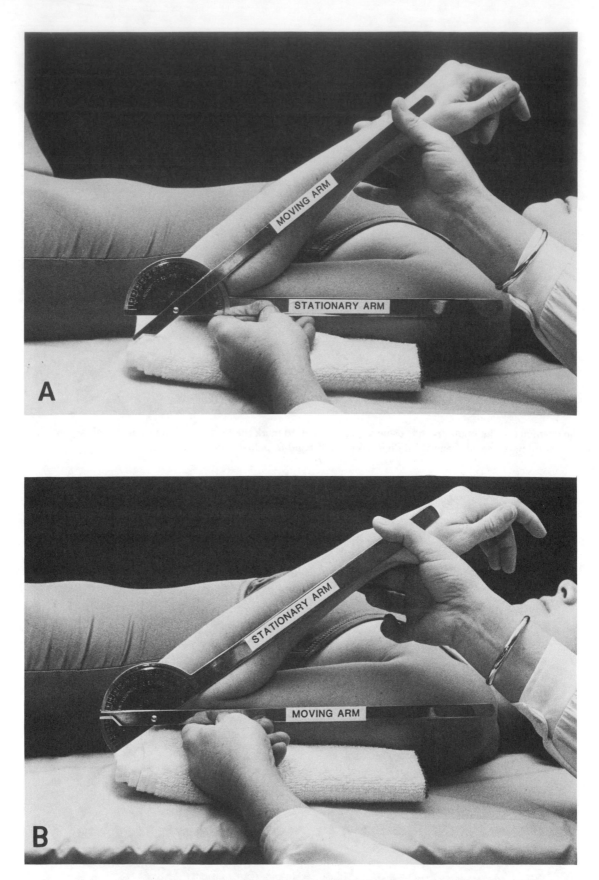

FIGURE 2-9. *A,* When a half-circle goniometer is used to measure the subject's left elbow flexion, alignment of the moving arm with the subject's forearm causes the pointer to move beyond the body of the goniometer and therefore makes it impossible to read the scale on the body. *B,* If the arms of the goniometer are reversed so that the stationary arm is aligned parallel to the moving part and the moving arm is aligned parallel to the proximal part, the pointer remains on the body of the goniometer and the scale may be read along the pointer.

MEASUREMENT OF JOINT MOTION: A GUIDE TO GONIOMETRY

the joint. The term DISTAL ARM will be used to refer to the arm aligned with the distal portion of the joint. The ANATOMIC LANDMARKS provide reference points that help to insure that the alignment of the arms is correct.

The FULCRUM of the goniometer should be placed over the approximate location of the axis of motion of the joint being measured. Because the axis of motion may change during movement, the location of the fulcrum must be adjusted accordingly. Moore[1] suggests that careful alignment of the proximal and distal arms insures that the fulcrum of the goniometer will be located at the approximate axis of motion. Therefore, alignment of the arms of the goniometer should receive more emphasis than placement of the fulcrum over the axis of motion of the joint.

EXERCISE 3. GONIOMETER ALIGNMENT FOR ELBOW FLEXION

The following activities are designed to help the reader learn how to manipulate the goniometer.
Equipment: Full-circle and half-circle goniometers of plastic and metal in various sizes and a skin-marking pencil.
Activities:
1. Select a goniometer and a partner.
2. Position your partner so that he or she is supine. Your partner's right arm should be positioned so that it is close to the side of the body with the forearm in supination (palm of hand faces the ceiling). A pad placed under the humerus helps to insure that the elbow is fully extended.
3. Locate and mark each of the following landmarks with the pencil: acromion process, lateral epicondyle of the humerus, and the radial styloid process.
4. Align the proximal arm of the goniometer so that it parallels the longitudinal axis of the humerus, using the acromion process and the lateral epicondyle as reference points. Make sure that you are positioned so that the goniometer arm is at eye level during the alignment process.
5. Align the distal arm of the goniometer so that it parallels the longitudinal axis of the radius, using the lateral epicondyle of the humerus and the radial styloid process as landmarks.
6. Check the fulcrum to make sure that it is located over the lateral epicondyle. Also, check to make sure that the body of the goniometer is not being deflected by the supporting surface.
7. Recheck the alignment of the proximal arm and realign as necessary.
8. Read the scale on the goniometer and remove the instrument from the subject's arm.
9. Move the subject's forearm into various positions in the flexion ROM, including the end of the flexion ROM. At each joint position in the flexion ROM, align and read the goniometer. Remember that you must support the subject's forearm while aligning the goniometer.
10. Repeat steps 3 through 9 on the subject's upper left extremity.
11. Repeat steps 4 through 9 using goniometers of different sizes and shapes.
12. Answer the following questions:
Did the length of the goniometer arms affect the accuracy of the alignment? Explain.
What length goniometer arms would you recommend as being the most appropriate for this measurement? Why?
Did the type of goniometer used (full-circle and half-circle) affect either alignment or reading the scale? Explain.
Did the side of the body that you were testing make a difference in your ability to align the goniometer? Why?

RECORDING

The next step in learning how to use a goniometer is to learn how to record. Recordings should provide enough information to permit an accurate interpretation of the measurement. The following format for recording provides complete information and therefore has been adopted for use in this text. However, the reader should be aware of the fact that both the methods and forms used for recording goniometric measurements differ considerably among facilities.

RECOMMENDED ITEMS TO BE INCLUDED IN RECORDING

1. Subject's name, age, and sex
2. Examiner's name
3. Date and time of measurement
4. Location of measurement
5. Make and type of goniometer used
6. Range of motion: including the number of degrees at the beginning of the motion and the number of degrees at the end of the motion and the total range of motion.
7. Any subjective information, such as discomfort or pain, that is reported by the subject during the testing.
8. Any objective information obtained by the examiner during testing, such as the appearance of protective muscle spasm.
9. The type of goniometry performed, that is, passive or active motion.
10. A complete description of any deviation from the recommended testing positions.

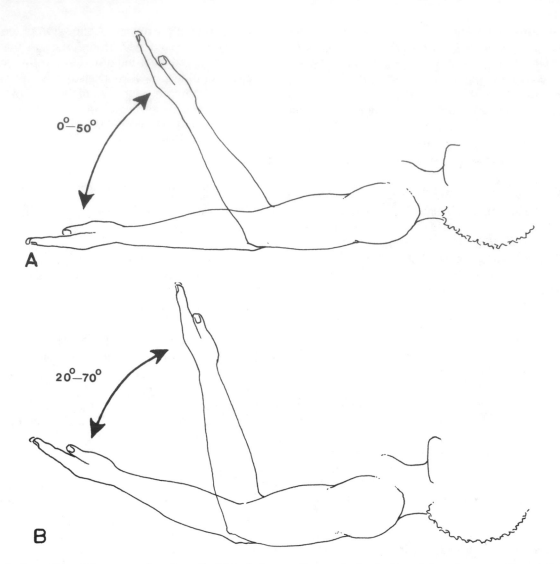

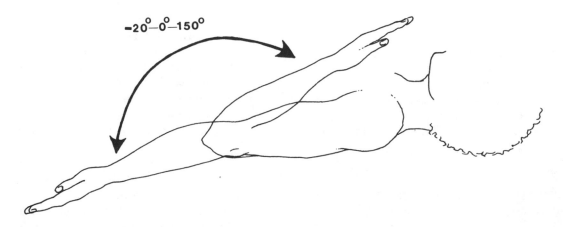

FIGURE 2-10. *A,* Recording of the range of motion should include a reading at the beginning of the range as well as at the end. In this illustration, the range of motion begins at 0 degrees and ends at 50 degrees, so the total range of motion is 50 degrees. *B,* In this subject the range of motion begins at 20 degrees of flexion and ends at 70 degrees; the total range of motion for this subject and the subject in part *A* is 50 degrees. However, two different arcs of motion are represented by the total number of degrees.

FIGURE 2-11. This subject has 20 degrees of hyperextension at her elbow. Therefore, the motion begins at −20 degrees and proceeds through the 0 position to 150 degrees.

Recordings should include the starting and ending positions to define the ROM. A recording that includes only the total ROM, such as 50 degrees of flexion, gives no information regarding where a motion begins and ends. Likewise, a recording that lists − 20 degrees of flexion is open to misinterpretation, because the lack of flexion could occur at either the end or the beginning of the ROM. The methods of recording described in the following sections are designed to provide a sufficient amount of information for accurate interpretation.

A motion, such as flexion, that begins at 0 and ends at 50 degrees of flexion is recorded as 0–50 degrees (Fig. 2-10A). A motion that begins with the joint flexed at 20 degrees and ends at 70 degrees of flexion is recorded as 20–70 degrees (Fig. 2-10B). The total ROM is the same (50 degrees) in both instances; but in the first instance, the motion begins at 0, while in the second instance, the motion begins at 20 degrees of flexion.

Because both the starting and ending positions have been recorded, the measurement can be interpreted correctly. The subject who has a 0–50 degree flexion ROM lacks motion at the end of the flexion ROM and is unable to complete the ROM. The subject with a 20–70 degree flexion ROM lacks the first portion of the flexion ROM and is unable to attain a zero starting position. The term hypomobile may be applied to these joints, because both joints have a less than normal range of motion.

Sometimes the opposite situation exists in which a joint has a greater-than-normal range of motion and is hypermobile. If an elbow joint is hypermobile, the starting position for measuring elbow flexion may be in hyperextension rather than at 0 degrees. If the elbow were hyperextended 20 degrees in the starting position, the beginning of the ROM would be recorded as − 20 degrees (Fig. 2-11). A range of motion that begins at 20 degrees of hyperextension and ends at 105 degrees of flexion is recorded as − 20−0−150 degrees. Inclusion of the zero starting position in the recording as well as the minus sign in front of the 20 degrees indicates that the range of motion begins at 20 degrees of hyperextension.

Prior to beginning a goniometric evaluation the examiner needs to:

- determine which joints and motions need to be tested
- organize the testing sequence by body position
- gather the necessary equipment, such as goniometers, padding, and recording forms
- prepare an explanation of the procedure for the subject

PROCEDURES

EXPLANATION PROCEDURE

The steps listed below and the example that follows provide the reader with a suggested format for explaining goniometry to a subject. Layman's terms rather than technical terms are used in the example so that the subject can understand the procedure. During the explanation, the examiner should to establish a good rapport with the subject and enlist the subject's participation in the evaluation process. After reading the example, the reader should practice Exercise 4.

Steps:
1. Introduction and explanation of purpose
2. Explanation and demonstration of goniometer
3. Explanation and demonstration of anatomic landmarks
4. Explanation and demonstration of recommended testing positions
5. Explanation and demonstration of examiner's and subject's roles
6. Confirmation of subject's understanding

EXAMPLE: EXPLANATION OF GONIOMETRY

1. Introduction and Explanation of Purpose
INTRODUCTION: I am Jill Jones, a student (occupational title).
EXPLANATION: I am here to measure the amount of motion that you have at your joints, for example, how much motion you have at your elbow.
DEMONSTRATION: Jill flexes and extends her elbow so that the subject is able to observe a joint motion.
2. Explanation and Demonstration of Goniometer
EXPLANATION: The instrument that I will be using to obtain the measurements is called a goniometer. It is similar to a protractor, but it has two extensions called arms.
DEMONSTRATION: Jill shows the goniometer to the subject. She lets the subject hold the goniometer and encourages the subject to ask questions. Jill shows the subject how the goniometer is used by holding it next to her own elbow.
3. Explanation and Demonstration of Anatomic Landmarks
EXPLANATION: In order to obtain accurate measurements, I will need to identify a number of anatomic landmarks. These landmarks help me to align the arms of the goniometer. Because these landmarks are important, I may have to ask you to remove certain articles of clothing, such as your shirt or blouse. Also, I may have to use my fingers to locate some of the landmarks.
DEMONSTRATION: Jill shows subject an easily identified anatomic landmark such as the ulnar styloid process, and a less easily identified landmark that requires palpation such as the capitate.
4. Explanations and Demonstration of Recommended Testing Positions
EXPLANATION: A series of recommended testing positions have been established which help to make joint measurements easier and more accurate. Whenever possible, I would like you to assume these positions. I will be happy to help you get into a particular position. Please let me know if you need assistance.
DEMONSTRATION: Sitting and supine positions.

...n and Demonstration of Examiner's/Subject's

Passive Motion

...TION: I will move your arm and take a mea-
...should relax and let me do all of the work.
...measurements should not cause discomfort. Please let me know if you have any discomfort, and I will stop moving your arm.

DEMONSTRATION: Move subject's arm gently and slowly through a range of elbow flexion.

Active Motion

EXPLANATION: I will ask you to move your arm in exactly the same way that I just moved your arm.

DEMONSTRATION: Take subject's arm through a passive range of motion, then ask subject to perform the same motion.

6. Confirmation of Subject Understanding

Do you have any questions? Would you like me to show you any other measurements? Are you ready to begin?

EXERCISE 4. EXPLANATION OF GONIOMETRY

Practice the following six steps with a partner.
1. Introduce yourself and explain the purpose of goniometric testing. Demonstrate a joint range of motion on yourself.
2. Show the goniometer to your subject and demonstrate how it is used to measure a joint ROM.
3. Explain why bony landmarks must be located and palpated. Demonstrate how you would locate a bony landmark on yourself and explain why clothing may have to be removed.
4. Explain and demonstrate why changes in position may be required.
5. Explain the subject's role in the procedure. Explain and demonstrate your role in the procedure.
6. Obtain confirmation of the subject's understanding of your explanation.

TESTING PROCEDURE

The testing process is initiated after the explanation of goniometry has been given and the examiner is assured that the subject understands the nature of the testing process.

The testing procedure consists of the following twelve-step sequence of activities. Exercise 5, which is based on the sequence, affords the reader an opportunity to use the testing procedure for an evaluation of the elbow joint. This exercise should be practiced until the examiner is able to perform the activities sequentially without reference to the exercise. When competency has been attained, the examiner should proceed to Exercises 6 and 7.

Twelve-Step Sequence
1. Place the subject in the recommended testing position.
2. Stabilize the proximal joint component.
3. Move the distal joint component through the available ROM. Make sure that the passive ROM is performed slowly and that the end of the range is attained and end-feel determined.
4. Make a clinical estimate of the ROM.
5. Return distal joint component to the starting position.
6. Palpate bony anatomic landmarks.
7. Align the goniometer.
8. Read and record the starting position. Remove goniometer.
9. Stabilize proximal joint component.
10. Move distal component through the full ROM.
11. Replace and realign goniometer.
12. Read and record ROM.

EXERCISE 5. TESTING PROCEDURE FOR GONIOMETRIC EVALUATION OF ELBOW FLEXION

1. Place the subject in a supine position with the arm to be tested positioned close to the side of the body. Place a pad under the distal end of the humerus to allow for full elbow extension. Position the forearm in full supination with the palm of the hand facing the ceiling.
2. Stabilize the distal end of the humerus to prevent flexion of the shoulder.
3. Move the forearm through the full passive range of flexion. Usually the end-feel is soft because of compression of the muscle bulk on the anterior forearm with that on the anterior humerus.
4. Make a clinical estimate of the total range of motion.
5. Return the forearm to the starting position.
6. Palpate bony landmarks (acromion process, lateral condyle of the humerus, and the radial styloid process) and mark with a skin pencil.
7. Align the fulcrum and arms of the goniometer.
   Place the fulcrum over the lateral condyle of the humerus.
   Align the proximal arm with the lateral midline of the humerus, using the acromion process for reference.
   Align the distal arm along the lateral midline of the radius, using the styloid process of the radius for reference.

8. Read the goniometer and record the starting position. Remove goniometer.
9. Stabilize the proximal joint component (humerus).
10. Perform the passive ROM making sure that you complete the available range.
11. When the end of the ROM has been attained, replace and re-align the goniometer.
12. Read the goniometer and record your reading. Compare your reading with your clinical estimate to make sure that you are reading the correct scale.

EXERCISE 6. INTRATESTER RELIABILITY

1. Select a partner and a goniometer.
2. Following the steps outlined in Exercise 4, perform three successive goniometeric measurements of elbow flexion on your partner.
3. Record each measurement on the recording form.
4. Compare the measurements. If a discrepancy of more than 5 degrees exists between measurements, recheck each step in the procedure to make sure that you are performing the steps correctly, and then repeat this exercise.
5. Continue practicing until you have obtained three successive measurements that are within 5 degrees of each other.
6. Repeat this exercise with other joints and motions.

RECORDING FORM FOR INTRATESTER RELIABILITY

Subject's Name _____ Age _____ Sex _____
Examiner's Name _____
Date _____ Time _____ Location _____
Type and Make of Goniometer _____
Type of Motion: Active _____ Passive _____

	LEFT	JOINT AND MOTIONS	RIGHT	COMMENTS
Test 1		Elbow Flexion		
Test 2				
Test 3				
Average				
Test 1		Knee Flexion		
Test 2				
Test 3				
Average				
Test 1				
Test 2				
Test 3				
Average				
Test 1				
Test 2				
Test 3				
Average				
Test 1				
Test 2				
Test 3				
Average				

EXERCISE 7. INTERTESTER RELIABILITY

1. Select a partner and a goniometer.
2. Measure the elbow flexion ROM on your subject following the steps outlined in Exercise 5.
3. Ask three examiners to measure the same elbow flexion ROM on your subject, using your goniometer and following the steps outlined in Exercise 5.
4. Record each measurement on the recording form.
5. Compare all measurements. If discrepancies between measurements are greater than 5 degrees, repeat the exercise. The examiners should observe one another's measurements to discover differences in technique that might account for variability, for example, faulty alignment, lack of stabilization, or reading the wrong scale.
6. Repeat this exercise with other joints and motions after you have learned the testing procedures.
7. Repeat this exercise using different goniometers.

RECORDING FORM FOR INTERTESTER RELIABILITY

Subject's Name _____ Age _____ Sex _____
Examiner #1 _____
Examiner #2 _____
Examiner #3 _____
Date _____ Time _____ Location _____
Type and Make of Goniometer _____
Type of Motion: Active _____ Passive _____

	LEFT	JOINT AND MOTIONS	RIGHT	COMMENTS
Examiner 1		Elbow Flexion		
Examiner 2				
Examiner 3				
Average				
Examiner 1		Knee Flexion		
Examiner 2				
Examiner 3				
Average				
Examiner 1				
Examiner 2				
Examiner 3				
Average				
Examiner 1				
Examiner 2				
Examiner 3				
Average				

UPPER EXTREMITY TESTING

OBJECTIVES

Upon completion of this chapter the reader will be able to:

1. Identify:
   the appropriate planes and axes for each upper extremity joint motion
   the structures that limit the end of the ROM at each upper extremity joint and the expected normal end-feel

2. Describe:
   the recommended testing positions used for each upper extremity joint motion

3. Perform a goniometric evaluation of any upper extremity joint including:
   a clear explanation of the testing procedure
   positioning of the subject in a recommended testing position
   adequate stabilization of the proximal joint component
   a correct determination of the end of the range of motion
   a correct identification of the end-feel
   palpation of the correct bony landmarks
   accurate alignment of the goniometer
   correct reading and recording

4. Plan a goniometric evaluation of the upper extremities that is organized by body position.

5. Assess intratester and intertester reliability of goniometric testing of upper extremity joints.

The recommended testing positions, stabilization techniques, physiologic end-feel, and goniometer alignment for the joints of the upper and lower extremities and the spine are presented in the following chapters. The goniometric evaluation should follow the twelve-step sequence that was presented in Exercise 5 of Chapter 2.

THE SHOULDER: GLENOHUMERAL JOINT/SHOULDER COMPLEX

Shoulder motion occurs at the glenohumeral, scapulothoracic, sternoclavicular, and acromioclavicular joints. Two methods of measuring the ROM of the shoulder may be used. One method restricts motion to the glenohumeral joint and measures only glenohumeral motion. This method is used to evaluate the integrity of the glenohumeral joint. The second method allows scapulothoracic, sternoclavicular, and acromioclavicular motion to occur along with glenohumeral motion. This method may be useful in evaluating the functional ability of the shoulder complex. Both methods of measuring the ROM of the shoulder are presented in the discussions of stabilization techniques and end-feels.

FLEXION

Motion occurs in the sagittal plane around a coronal axis.

RECOMMENDED TESTING POSITION

Position the subject supine with the knees flexed to flatten the lumbar spine. The shoulder is positioned in 0 degrees of abduction, adduction, and rotation. The forearm is posi-

tioned in 0 degrees of supination and pronation so that the palm of the hand faces the body.

STABILIZATION

Glenohumeral Motion (Fig. 3-1). Stabilize the scapula to prevent elevation, posterior tilting, and upward rotation of the scapula.

Shoulder Complex Motion. Stabilize the thorax to prevent extension of the spine.

PHYSIOLOGIC END-FEEL

Glenohumeral Motion. The end-feel is firm because of tension in the posterior band of the coracohumeral ligament, the posterior joint capsule, and the teres minor, teres major, and infraspinatus muscles.

Shoulder Complex Motion. The end-feel is firm because of tension in the latissimus dorsi muscle and the costosternal fibers of the pectoralis major muscle.

GONIOMETER ALIGNMENT (Figs. 3-2 and 3-3)

1. Center the fulcrum of the goniometer close to the acromion process.
2. Align the proximal arm with the mid-axillary line of the thorax.
3. Align the distal arm with the lateral midline of the humerus, using the lateral epicondyle of the humerus for reference.

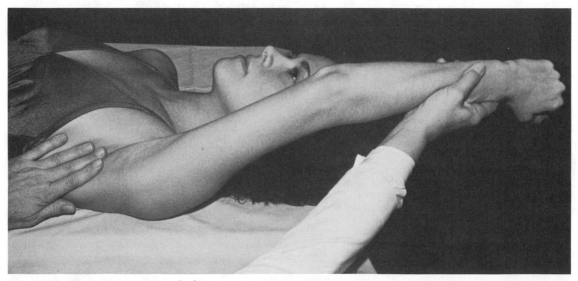

FIGURE 3-1. The subject's left upper extremity is shown at the end of the ROM of glenohumeral flexion. The examiner's left hand, which is placed over the lateral border of the subject's scapula, is the stabilizing hand. The examiner is able to determine that the end of the ROM has been reached, because any attempt to move the extremity into additional flexion causes the lateral border of the scapula to move anteriorly and laterally. The stabilizing hand detects and prevents scapular motion.

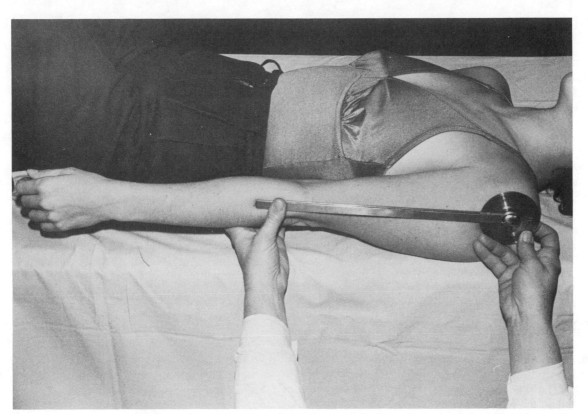

FIGURE 3-2. The subject is shown at the beginning of the ROM of glenohumeral flexion. The body of the full-circle metal goniometer is aligned with the subject's acromion process. The two arms of the goniometer are aligned along the lateral midline of the thorax and the lateral midline of the humerus and extend over the lateral epicondyle of the humerus.

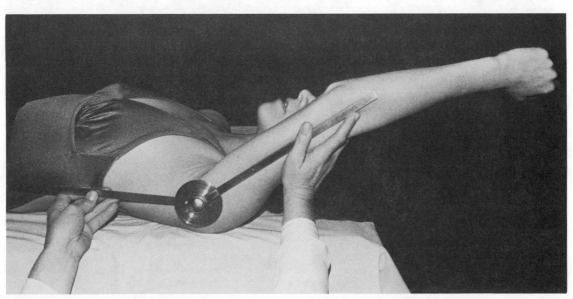

FIGURE 3-3. This photograph illustrates the alignment of the goniometer at the end of the ROM of glenohumeral flexion. The examiner's right hand supports the subject's extremity and maintains the goniometer's distal arm in correct alignment over the lateral epicondyle. The examiner's left hand aligns the goniometer's proximal arm with the lateral midline of the thorax.

EXTENSION

Motion occurs in the sagittal plane around a coronal axis.

RECOMMENDED TESTING POSITION

Position the subject prone with the head facing away from the shoulder being tested. No pillow is used under the head. The shoulder is positioned in 0 degrees of abduction and rotation. The elbow is positioned in slight flexion so that tension in the long head of the biceps brachii muscle will not restrict the motion. The forearm is positioned in 0 degrees of supination and pronation so that the palm of the hand faces the body.

STABILIZATION

Glenohumeral Motion (Fig. 3-4). Stabilize the scapula to prevent elevation and anterior tilting (inferior angle protrudes posteriorly) of the scapula.

Shoulder Complex Motion. Stabilize the thorax to prevent forward flexion of the spine.

PHYSIOLOGIC END-FEEL

Glenohumeral Motion. The end-feel is firm because of tension in the anterior band of the coracohumeral ligament and the anterior joint capsule.

Shoulder Complex Motion. The end-feel is firm because of tension in the clavicular fibers of the pectoralis major muscle and the serratus anterior muscle.

GONIOMETER ALIGNMENT (Figs. 3-5 and 3-6)

1. Center the fulcrum of the goniometer close to the acromion process.
2. Align the proximal arm with the mid-axillary line of the thorax.
3. Align the distal arm with the lateral midline of the humerus, using the lateral epicondyle of the humerus for reference.

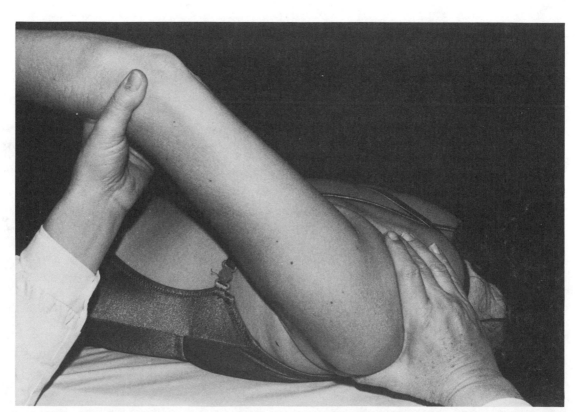

FIGURE 3-4. The subject's right upper extremity is shown at the end of the ROM of extension. The examiner's right hand is grasping the scapula. The examiner is able to determine that the end of the ROM in extension has been attained because additional extension causes the scapula to elevate and tilt anteriorly. The examiner's stabilizing hand detects and prevents scapular motion.

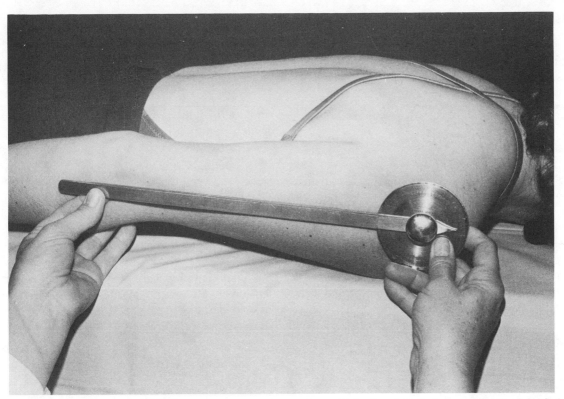

FIGURE 3-5. The subject is shown in the beginning of the ROM of extension with her head turned away from the joint being tested. The body of the goniometer is aligned with the acromion process, and the arms are aligned along the lateral midline of the thorax and the lateral midline of the humerus and extend over the lateral epicondyle.

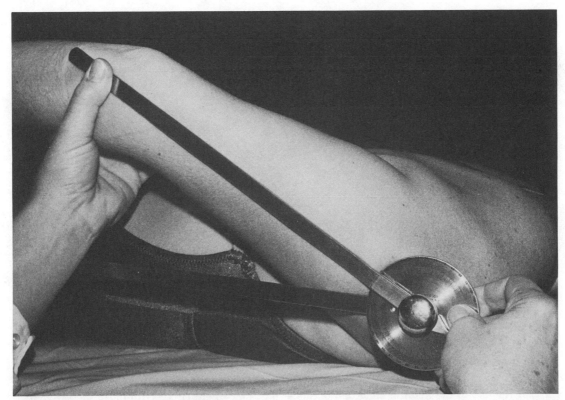

FIGURE 3-6. This photograph shows the goniometer alignment at the end of the ROM in extension. The examiner's left hand supports the subject's extremity and holds the distal arm of the goniometer in correct alignment over the lateral epicondyle of the humerus. The goniometer body is held over the subject's acromion process, while the proximal arm is aligned along the lateral midline of the thorax.

ABDUCTION

Motion occurs in the frontal plane around an anterior-posterior axis.

RECOMMENDED TESTING POSITION

Position the subject supine. As an alternative, measurements may be taken with the subject sitting or prone. The shoulder is positioned in 0 degrees of flexion and extension and full lateral rotation so that the palm of the hand faces anteriorly. If the humerus is not laterally rotated, contact between the greater tubercle of the humerus and the upper portion of the glenoid fossa or acromion process will restrict the motion. The elbow should be extended so that tension in the long head of the triceps will not restrict the motion.

STABILIZATION

Glenohumeral Motion (Figs. 3-7 and 3-8). Stabilize the scapula to prevent upward rotation and elevation of the scapula. Figure 3-8 shows an alternative method.

Shoulder Complex Motion. Stabilize the thorax to prevent lateral flexion of the spine.

PHYSIOLOGIC END-FEEL

Glenohumeral Motion. The end-feel is usually firm because of tension in the middle and inferior bands of the glenohumeral ligament, the inferior joint capsule, and the latissimus dorsi and pectoralis major muscles.

Shoulder Complex Motion. The end-feel is firm because of tension in the rhomboid major muscle, rhomboid minor muscle, and the middle and inferior portion of the trapezius muscle.

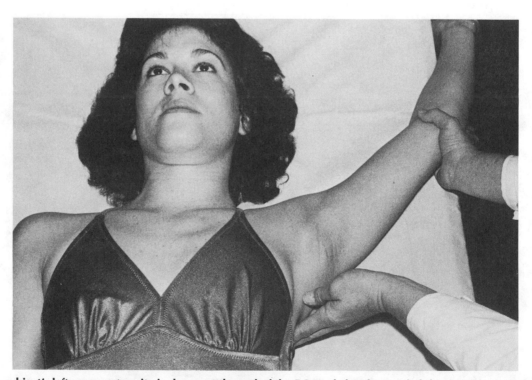

FIGURE 3-7. The subject's left upper extremity is shown at the end of the ROM of glenohumeral abduction. The examiner's left hand is stabilizing the scapula. The end of the ROM in abduction occurs at the point where attempts to move the extremity into additional abduction result in lateral scapular motion. This scapular motion may be detected by the stabilizing hand. The supine testing position is somewhat easier to use than the alternative sitting position, because in the supine position the subject's extremity and trunk are supported by the table.

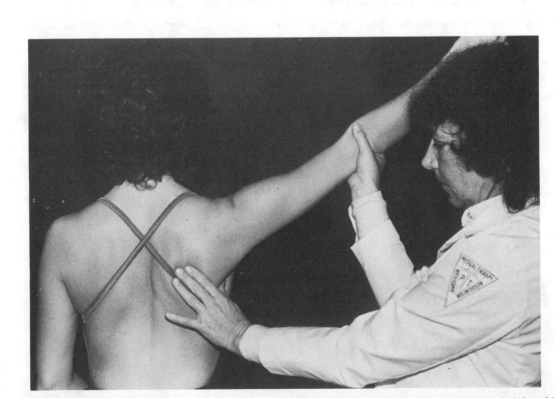

FIGURE 3-8. The subject's right upper extremity is shown at the end of the ROM in abduction. The examiner's left hand is stabilizing the scapula. The end of the ROM in abduction occurs when additional motion of the extremity causes the inferior angle of the scapula to move laterally away from the rib cage. The examiner's left hand is able to detect the lateral scapular motion. In the sitting position, the trunk is not as well stabilized as it is in the supine position; therefore, the examiner must be alert for lateral bending of the thorax. Also the subject may be asked to try to keep her back straight.

GONIOMETER ALIGNMENT (Supine Position)
(Figs. 3-9 and 3-10)

1. Center the fulcrum of the goniometer close to the anterior aspect of the acromion process.

2. Align the proximal arm so that it is parallel to the midline of the anterior aspect of the sternum.

3. At the end of the ROM, align the distal arm with the medial midline of the humerus, using the medial epicondyle for reference.

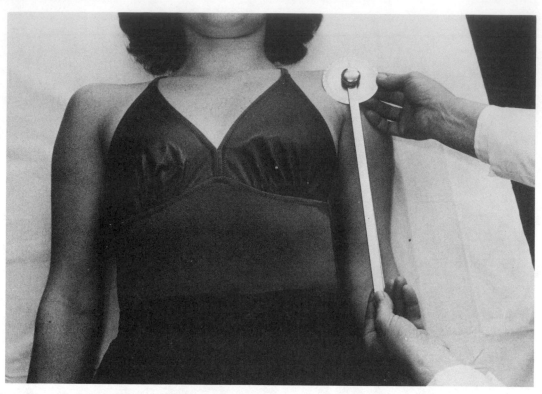

FIGURE 3-9. The supine starting position for abduction shows the body of the goniometer aligned over the anterior aspect of the acromion process. The arms of the goniometer are aligned along the anterior midline of the humerus and parallel to the sternum.

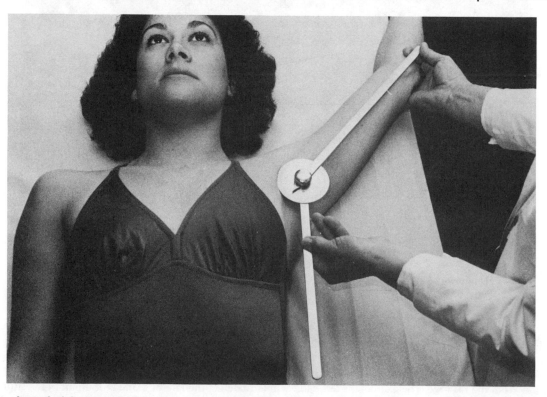

FIGURE 3-10. At the end of the ROM in abduction, the proximal arm of the goniometer is aligned parallel to the sternum. The distal arm of the goniometer is held in position along the medial midline of the humerus by the examiner. Note that the humerus is laterally rotated.

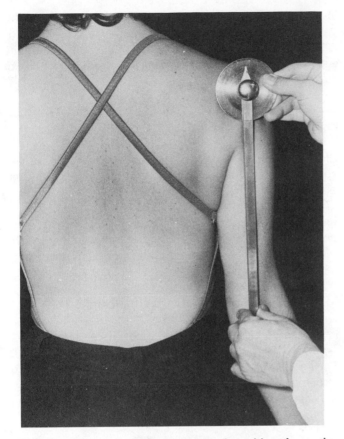

ALTERNATIVE GONIOMETER ALIGNMENT
(Sitting Position) (Figs. 3-11 and 3-12)

1. Center the fulcrum of the goniometer close to the posterior aspect of the acromion process.
2. Align the proximal arm parallel to the spinous processes of the vertebral column.
3. At the end of the ROM, align the distal arm with the lateral midline of the humerus, using the lateral epicondyle for reference.

ADDUCTION

Motion occurs in the frontal plane around an anterior-posterior axis.

RECOMMENDED TESTING POSITION, STABILIZATION, AND GONIOMETER ALIGNMENT

The testing position, stabilization, and alignment are the same as for shoulder abduction.

FIGURE 3-11. The body of the goniometer is positioned over the posterior aspect of the acromion process when measuring abduction in the sitting position. The two arms of the goniometer are aligned along the posterior midline of the humerus and parallel to the spinous processes of the vertebral column.

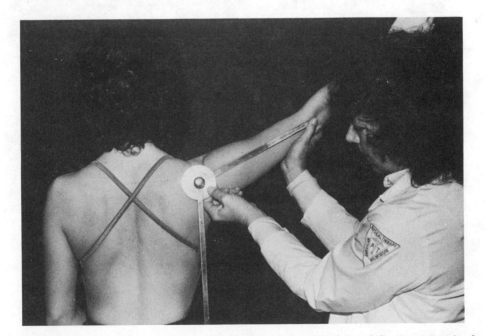

FIGURE 3-12. This photograph shows the alignment of the goniometer at the end of the abduction ROM in the sitting position. The examiner's right hand supports the subject's right upper extremity and holds the distal arm of the goniometer aligned along the lateral midline of the humerus. The proximal arm should be free to hang perpendicularly to the floor and parallel to the subject's vertebral column. Sometimes the sitting position is more awkward than the supine position, because the weight of the subject's extremity must be supported by the examiner during passive ROM and the subject's thorax must be watched constantly to make sure that no lateral flexion is occurring.

MEDIAL (INTERNAL) ROTATION

Motion occurs in the transverse plane around a longitudinal axis when the subject is in anatomic position.

RECOMMENDED TESTING POSITION

Position the subject supine, with the arm being tested in 90 degrees of shoulder abduction. The forearm is perpendicular to the supporting surface and is in 0 degrees of supination and pronation so that the palm of the hand faces the feet. The full length of the humerus rests on the supporting surface. The elbow is not supported. A pad is placed under the humerus so that the humerus is positioned level with the acromion process.

STABILIZATION

Glenohumeral Motion (Fig. 3-13). In the beginning of the ROM, stabilization is often needed at the distal end of the humerus to keep the shoulder in 90 degrees of abduction. Toward the end of the ROM, the scapula is stabilized to prevent elevation and anterior tilting (inferior angle protrudes posteriorly) of the scapula.

Shoulder Complex Motion. In the beginning of the ROM, stabilization is often needed at the distal end of the humerus to keep the shoulder in 90 degrees of abduction. Toward the end of the ROM the thorax is stabilized to prevent flexion of the spine.

PHYSIOLOGIC END-FEEL

Glenohumeral Motion. The end-feel is firm because of tension in the posterior joint capsule and the infraspinatus and teres minor muscles.

Shoulder Complex Motion. The end-feel is firm because of tension in the rhomboid major and minor muscles, and the middle and inferior portions of the trapezius muscle.

GONIOMETER ALIGNMENT (Figs. 3-14 and 3-15)

1. Center the fulcrum of the goniometer over the olecranon process.
2. Align the proximal arm so that it is either parallel to or perpendicular to the floor.
3. Align the distal arm with the ulna, using the olecranon process and ulnar styloid for reference.

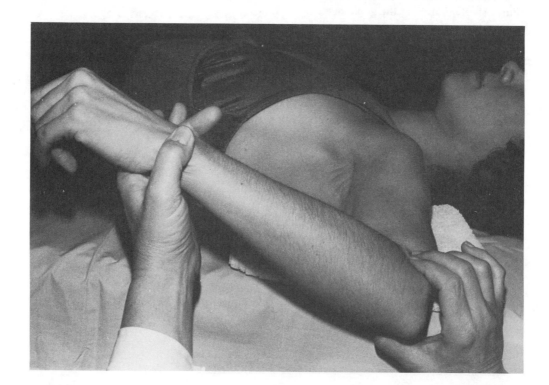

FIGURE 3-13. The subject's left upper extremity is shown at the end of the ROM of medial (internal) rotation of the shoulder. The glenohumeral joint is positioned at 90 degrees of abduction, and the elbow is maintained in 90 degrees of flexion. The examiner's right hand is stabilizing at the distal end of the humerus to maintain the abducted shoulder position. The end of the ROM in medial rotation occurs when continuation of the motion causes the scapula to tilt anteriorly. The scapular motion may be observed at the anterior and superior aspect of the shoulder.

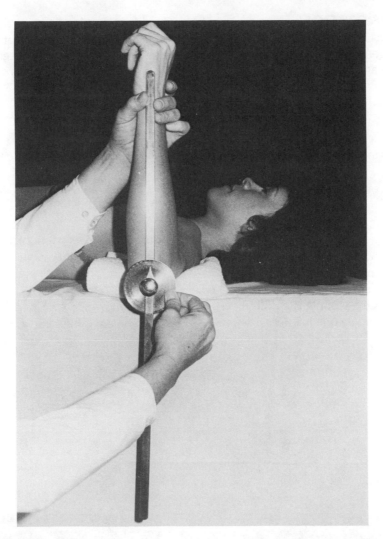

FIGURE 3-14. The body of the goniometer is placed over the olecranon process, and the distal arm is aligned with the ulnar styloid process in the testing positions for both medial and lateral rotation at the glenohumeral joint. The proximal arm of the goniometer should be freely movable so that gravitational force will position the arm perpendicular to the floor.

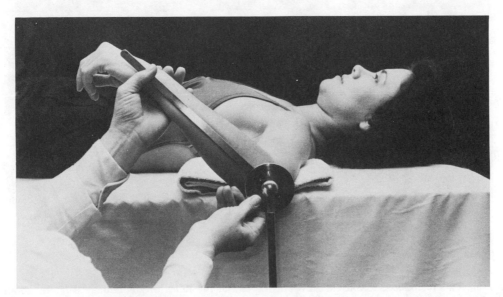

FIGURE 3-15. The examiner is supporting the subject's left forearm and maintaining the distal arm of the goniometer over the ulnar styloid process at the end of the ROM of medial rotation. The examiner's right hand is holding the body of the goniometer over the olecranon process. The proximal arm of the goniometer is freely movable and should hang so that it is perpendicular to the floor.

LATERAL (EXTERNAL) ROTATION

Motion occurs in the transverse plane around a longitudinal axis when the subject is in anatomic position.

RECOMMENDED TESTING POSITION

The testing position is the same as for medial rotation of the shoulder.

STABILIZATION

Glenohumeral Motion (Fig. 3-16). In the beginning of the ROM, stabilization is often needed at the distal end of the humerus to keep the shoulder in 90 degrees of abduction. Toward the end of the ROM the scapula is stabilized to prevent posterior tilting of the scapula (the inferior angle presses against the rib cage).

Shoulder Complex Motion. In the beginning of the ROM, stabilization is often needed at the distal end of the humerus to keep the shoulder in 90 degrees of abduction. Toward the end of the ROM the thorax is stabilized to prevent extension of the spine.

PHYSIOLOGIC END-FEEL

Glenohumeral Motion. The end-feel is firm because of tension in the three bands of the glenohumeral ligament, the coracohumeral ligament, the anterior joint capsule, and the subscapularis, pectoralis major, latissimus dorsi, and teres major muscles.

Shoulder Complex Motion. The end-feel is firm because of tension in the serratus anterior and pectoralis minor muscles.

GONIOMETER ALIGNMENT (Figs. 3-17 and 3-18)

The alignment is the same as for medial rotation of the shoulder.

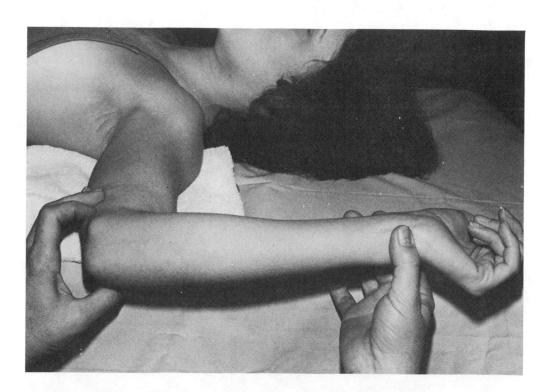

FIGURE 3-16. The subject's left upper extremity is shown at the end of the ROM of glenohumeral lateral rotation. The examiner is stabilizing the distal humerus to prevent abduction beyond 90 degrees. The examiner uses his right hand to move the forearm while preventing either supination or elbow extension. The end of the ROM in lateral rotation is attained when additional motion causes the scapula to press against the posterior rib cage.

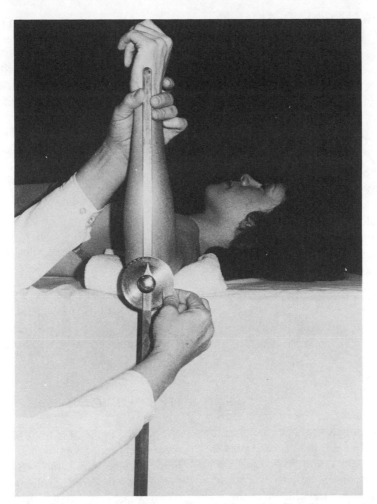

FIGURE 3-17. The goniometer alignment for ROM in lateral rotation is the same as the alignment for medial rotation. However, the examiner will need to change hand positions so that the left hand rather than the right hand holds the body of the goniometer as shown in Figure 3-18.

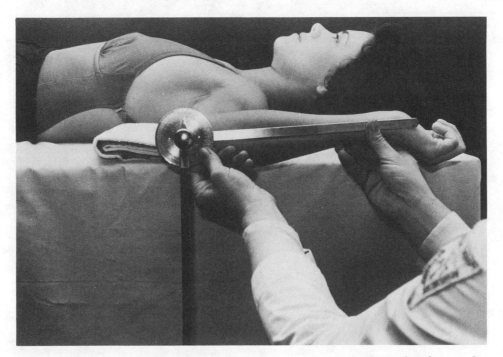

FIGURE 3-18. The alignment of the goniometer at the end of the ROM in lateral rotation shows that the examiner may need to sit on a chair or a stool in order to read the goniometer at eye level.

THE ELBOW: HUMEROULNAR AND HUMERORADIAL JOINTS

FLEXION

Motion occurs in the sagittal plane around a coronal axis.

RECOMMENDED TESTING POSITION

Position the subject supine with the shoulder positioned in 0 degrees of flexion, extension, and abduction so that the arm is close to the side of the body. A pad is placed under the distal end of the humerus to allow full elbow extension. The forearm is positioned in full supination with the palm of the hand facing the ceiling.

STABILIZATION (Fig. 3-19)

Stabilize the distal end of the humerus to prevent flexion of the shoulder.

PHYSIOLOGIC END-FEEL

Usually the end-feel is soft because of compression of the muscle bulk of the anterior forearm with that of the anterior upper arm. If the muscle bulk is small, the end-feel may be hard because of contact between the coronoid process of the ulna and coronoid fossa of the humerus, and contact between the head of the radius and the radial fossa of the hu-

merus. The end-feel may be firm because of tension in the posterior joint capsule and the triceps brachii muscle.

GONIOMETER ALIGNMENT (Figs. 3-20 and 3-21)

1. Center the fulcrum of the goniometer over the lateral epicondyle of the humerus.
2. Align the proximal arm with the lateral midline of the humerus, using the acromion process for reference.
3. Align the distal arm with the lateral midline of the radius, using the styloid process for reference.

EXTENSION

Motion occurs in the sagittal plane around a coronal axis.

RECOMMENDED TESTING POSITION, STABILIZATION, AND GONIOMETER ALIGNMENT

The testing position, stabilization, and alignment are the same as for elbow flexion.

PHYSIOLOGIC END-FEEL

Usually the end-feel is hard because of contact between the olecranon process of the ulna and the olecranon fossa of the humerus. Sometimes the end-feel is firm because of tension in the anterior joint capsule, the collateral ligaments, and the biceps brachii and brachialis muscles.

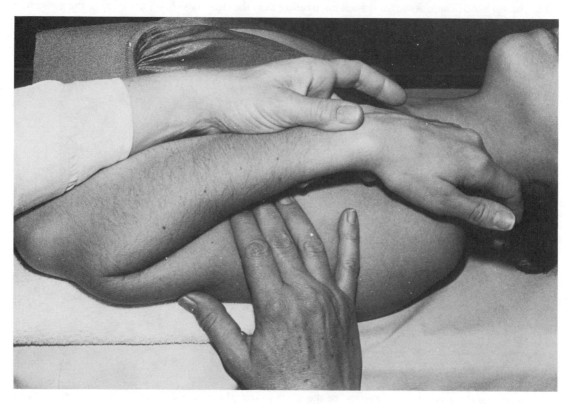

FIGURE 3-19. The photograph shows the end of the ROM of elbow flexion.

MEASUREMENT OF JOINT MOTION: A GUIDE TO GONIOMETRY

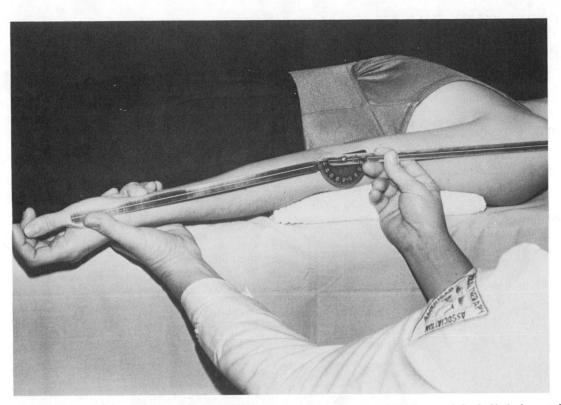

FIGURE 3-20. In the starting position for measuring the ROM for elbow flexion, the proximal arm of the half-circle metal goniometer is positioned along the lateral midline of the subject's left humerus. The distal arm of the goniometer is positioned along the lateral midline of the forearm and is aligned with the radial styloid process. A towel is placed under the distal humerus and elbow to ensure that the supporting surface does not prevent the full ROM of elbow extension. As can be seen in the photograph, the subject's elbow is in about 10 degrees of hyperextension; therefore, the ROM of elbow flexion begins at −10 degrees rather than at 0 degrees.

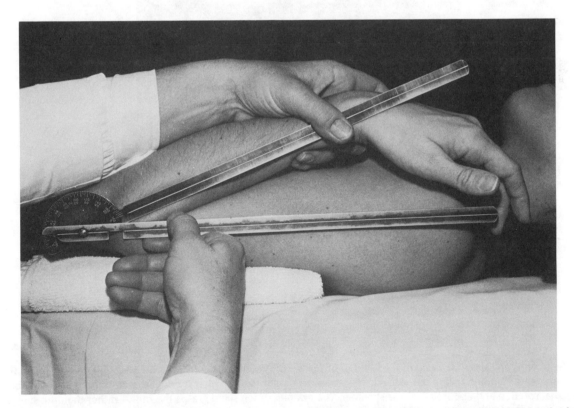

FIGURE 3-21. The examiner's left hand holds the distal arm of the goniometer aligned over the subject's left radial styloid process at the end of elbow flexion. The examiner's right hand is used to hold the proximal arm in alignment along the lateral midline of the subject's humerus.

THE FOREARM: RADIOULNAR JOINT

PRONATION

Motion occurs in the transverse plane around a longitudinal axis when the subject is in the anatomic position.

RECOMMENDED TESTING POSITION

Position the subject sitting with the shoulder in 0 degrees of flexion, extension, abduction, adduction, and rotation so that the upper arm is close to the side of the body. The elbow is flexed to 90 degrees, and the forearm is supported by the examiner. The forearm is initially positioned midway between supination and pronation so that the thumb points toward the ceiling.

STABILIZATION (Fig. 3-22)

Stabilize the distal end of the humerus to prevent medial rotation and abduction of the shoulder.

PHYSIOLOGIC END-FEEL

The end-feel is hard because of contact between the ulna and the radius, or it may be firm because of tension in the dorsal radioulnar ligament of the inferior radioulnar joint, the interosseous membrane, and the supinator and biceps brachii muscles.

GONIOMETER ALIGNMENT (Figs. 3-23 and 3-24)

1. Center the fulcrum of the goniometer lateral to the ulnar styloid process.
2. Align the proximal arm parallel to the anterior midline of the humerus.
3. Place the distal arm across the dorsal aspect of the forearm, just proximal to the styloid processes of the radius and ulna, where the forearm is most level and free of muscle bulk.

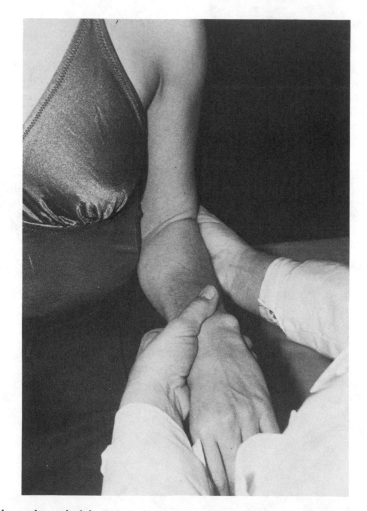

FIGURE 3-22. The photograph shows the end of the ROM of pronation of the subject's left forearm. The subject is sitting on the edge of a table and the examiner is standing facing the subject. The examiner's right hand, which is cupped around the subject's elbow, helps to prevent both medial rotation and abduction of the shoulder. The examiner's left hand grasps the radius rather than the subject's wrist or hand. If the examiner grasps either the subject's wrist or hand, movement of the wrist may be mistaken for movement at the radioulnar joints. The end of the ROM in pronation occurs when resistance prevents further motion from occurring at the forearm and medial rotation or abduction at the shoulder begins.

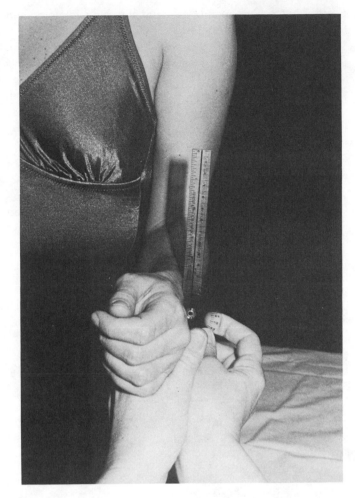

FIGURE 3-23. In the starting position for pronation, the goniometer is placed lateral to the distal radioulnar joints. The arms of the goniometer are aligned parallel to the anterior midline of the humerus.

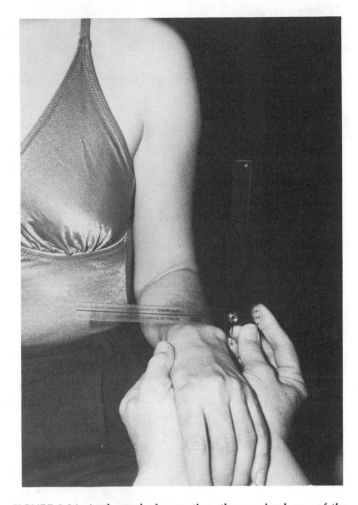

FIGURE 3-24. At the end of pronation, the proximal arm of the goniometer is aligned parallel to the anterior midline of the humerus, while the distal arm lies across the dorsum of the forearm just proximal to the radial and ulnar styloid processes. The fulcrum of the goniometer is aligned so that it is proximal and lateral to the ulnar styloid process.

SUPINATION

RECOMMENDED TESTING POSITION

The testing position is the same as for pronation of the forearm.

STABILIZATION (Fig. 3-25)

Stabilize the distal end of the humerus to prevent lateral rotation and adduction of the shoulder.

PHYSIOLOGIC END-FEEL

The end-feel is firm because of tension in the palmar radioulnar ligament of the inferior radioulnar joint, oblique cord, interosseous membrane, and the pronator teres and pronator quadratus muscles.

GONIOMETER ALIGNMENT (Figs. 3-26 and 3-27)

1. Center the goniometer medial to the ulnar styloid process.
2. Align the proximal arm parallel to the anterior midline of the humerus.
3. Place the distal arm across the ventral aspect of the forearm, just proximal to the styloid processes, where the forearm is most level and free of muscle bulk.

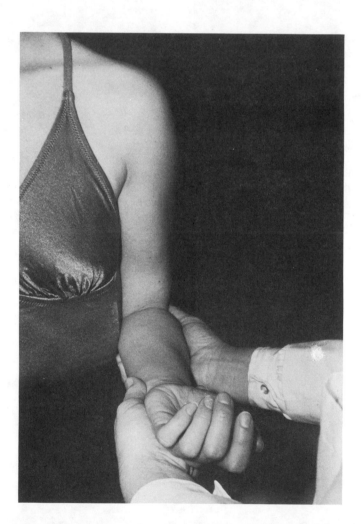

FIGURE 3-25. The photograph shows the subject's left forearm at the end of the ROM in supination. The examiner's right hand holds the elbow in close proximity to the subject's body and in 90 degrees of elbow flexion. The examiner's left hand, which is grasping the radius, also serves to support the forearm. The end of the supination ROM is attained when attempts to move the subject's forearm into additional supination meet with resistance and cause either adduction or lateral rotation at the shoulder.

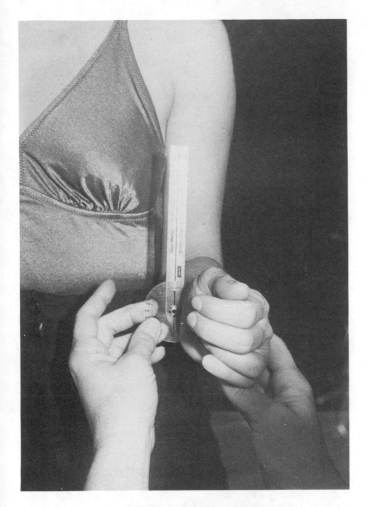

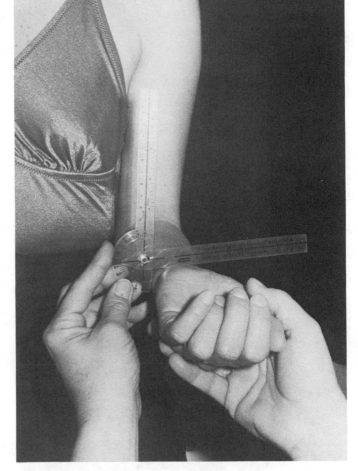

FIGURE 3-26. In the starting position for measuring the ROM in supination, the goniometer body is placed on the medial aspect of the forearm at the level of the distal radioulnar joints. The arms of the goniometer are aligned parallel to the anterior midline of the humerus. In the photograph, the examiner's right hand supports the subject's forearm and helps to keep the elbow at 90 degrees of flexion.

FIGURE 3-27. The goniometer alignment at the end of the ROM of supination shows that the distal arm of the goniometer rests on the medial aspect of the forearm at the level of the distal radioulnar joints. The position of the examiner's right hand is incorrect because it was altered for the photograph. The examiner's right hand should be grasping the subject's radius rather than the subject's hand.

THE WRIST: RADIOCARPAL AND INTERCARPAL JOINTS

FLEXION

Motion occurs in the sagittal plane around a coronal axis.

RECOMMENDED TESTING POSITION

Position the subject so that he or she is sitting next to a supporting surface. The shoulder is abducted to 90 degrees, and the elbow is flexed to 90 degrees. The forearm is positioned midway between supination and pronation so that the palm of the hand faces the ground. The forearm rests on the supporting surface, but the hand is free to move. Avoid radial or ulnar deviation of the wrist and flexion of the fingers. (If the fingers are flexed, tension in the extensor digitorum communis, extensor indicis, and extensor digiti minimi muscles will restrict the motion.)

STABILIZATION (Fig. 3-28)

Stabilize the radius and ulna to prevent supination or pronation of the forearm.

PHYSIOLOGIC END-FEEL

The end-feel is firm because of tension in the dorsal radiocarpal ligament and the dorsal joint capsule.

GONIOMETER ALIGNMENT (Figs. 3-29 and 3-30)

1. Center the fulcrum of the goniometer over the lateral aspect of the wrist close to the triquetrum.
2. Align the proximal arm with the lateral midline of the ulna, using the olecranon process for reference.
3. Align the distal arm with the lateral midline of the fifth metacarpal.

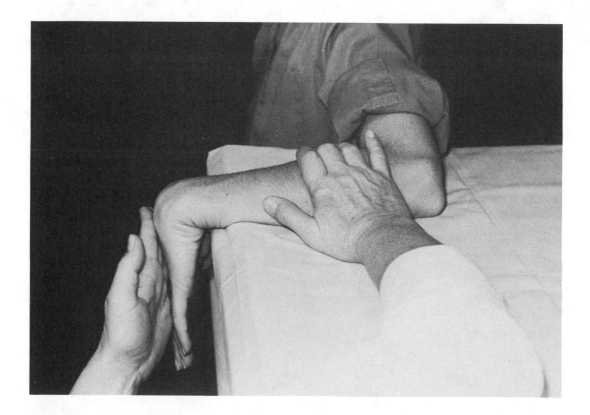

FIGURE 3-28. The photograph shows the end of wrist flexion (palmar flexion) ROM. The subject is seated on a low stool so that her humerus rests on the supporting surface when the glenohumeral joint is at 90 degrees of abduction. The subject's elbow is flexed at 90 degrees of flexion and about three-quarters of the subject's forearm is supported by the table. It is not possible to support the entire forearm because one needs to leave sufficient space for the hand to move freely. The examiner's hand exerts pressure over the dorsum of the hand to complete the ROM.

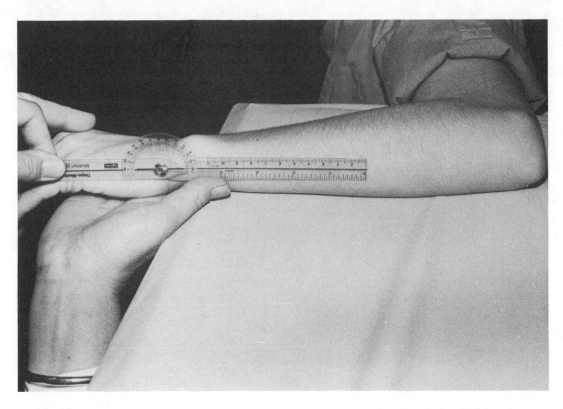

FIGURE 3-29. In the starting position for palmar flexion, the body of the goniometer is placed at the level of the triquetrum. The proximal goniometer arm is aligned along the ulna in line with the olecranon process. The distal goniometer arm is aligned along the fifth metacarpal.

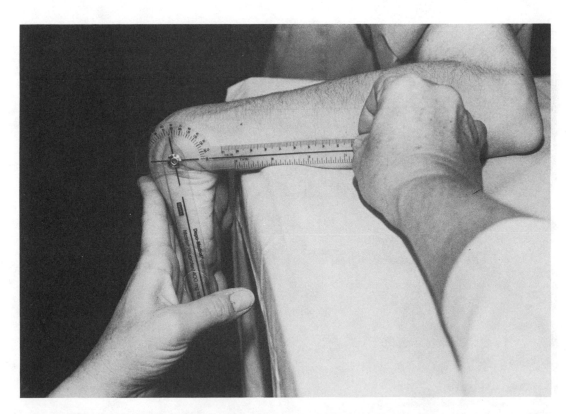

FIGURE 3-30. At the end of the ROM in palmar flexion the goniometer body lies over the lateral aspect of the carpal bones just distal to the ulnar styloid process. The distal goniometer arm is aligned with the subject's fifth metacarpal. The examiner maintains the wrist in palmar flexion by using her left hand to exert pressure on the middle dorsum of the subject's hand. The examiner avoids exerting pressure directly on the fifth metacarpal because such pressure will distort the goniometer alignment.

EXTENSION (Dorsal Flexion)

RECOMMENDED TESTING POSITION AND STABILIZATION (Fig. 3-31)

The testing position and stabilization are similar to those used when measuring wrist flexion. Avoid extension of the fingers so that tension in the flexor digitorum superficialis and profundus muscles will not restrict the motion.

PHYSIOLOGIC END-FEEL

Usually the end-feel is firm because of tension in the palmar radiocarpal ligament and the palmar joint capsule, but it may be hard because of contact between the radius and the carpal bones.

GONIOMETER ALIGNMENT (Figs. 3-32 and 3-33)

The alignment is the same as for wrist flexion.

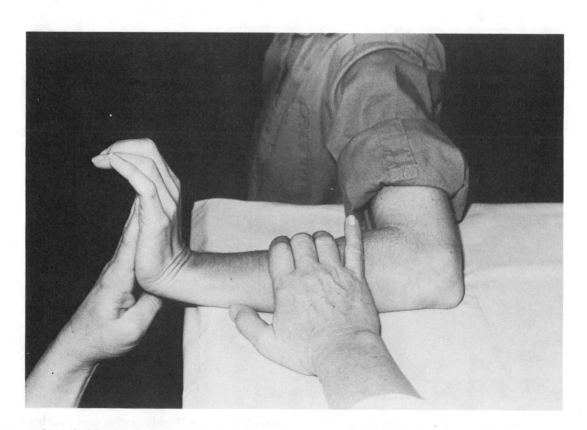

FIGURE 3-31. At the end of the wrist extension (dorsiflexion) ROM, the examiner's right hand stabilizes the subject's elbow at 90 degrees of flexion and helps to prevent lateral rotation at the subject's glenohumeral joint. The examiner's left hand holds the subject's left wrist in extension. The examiner is careful to distribute pressure equally across the subject's four metacarpals.

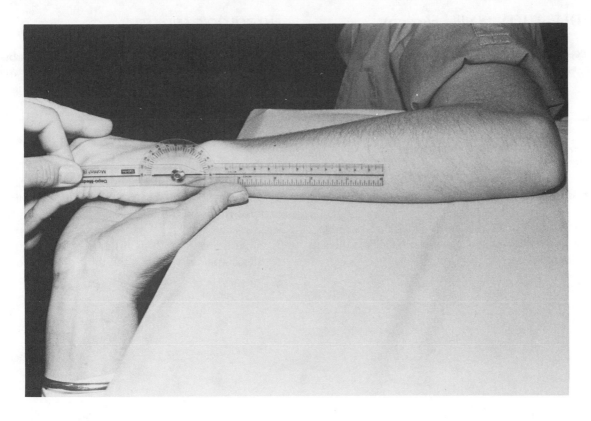

FIGURE 3-32. The starting position and goniometer alignment for wrist extension are the same as for measuring wrist palmar flexion.

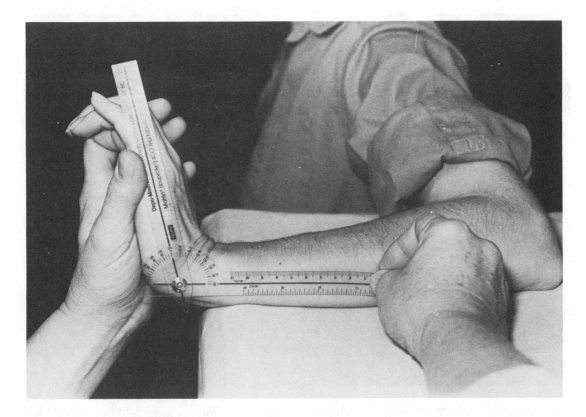

FIGURE 3-33. At the end of the ROM of wrist extension, the examiner's left hand maintains the alignment of the distal goniometer arm with the fifth metacarpal while at the same time holding the wrist in extension. The examiner avoids exerting excessive pressure on the fifth metacarpal.

RADIAL DEVIATION (Radial Flexion)

Motion occurs in the frontal plane around an anterior-posterior axis.

RECOMMENDED TESTING POSITION

The testing position is the same as for wrist flexion.

STABILIZATION (Fig. 3-34)

Stabilize the distal ends of the radius and ulna to prevent pronation or supination of the forearm and elbow flexion beyond 90 degrees.

PHYSIOLOGIC END-FEEL

Usually the end-feel is hard because of contact between the radial styloid process and the scaphoid, but it may be firm because of tension in the ulnar collateral ligament, ulnocarpal ligament, and ulnar portion of the joint capsule.

GONIOMETER ALIGNMENT (Figs. 3-35 and 3-36)

1. Center the fulcrum of the goniometer over the middle of the dorsal aspect of the wrist close to the capitate.
2. Align the proximal arm with the dorsal midline of the forearm, using the lateral epicondyle of the humerus for reference.
3. Align the distal arm with the dorsal midline of the third metacarpal. Do *not* use the third phalanx for reference.

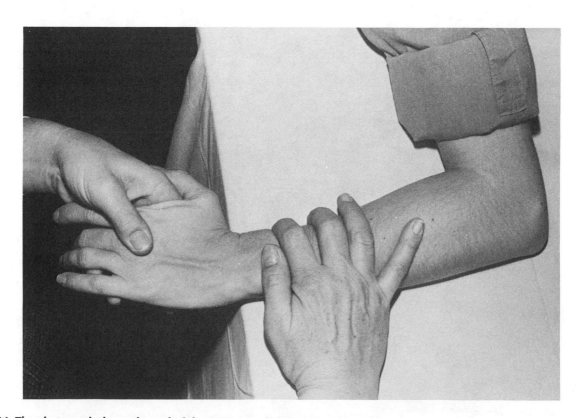

FIGURE 3-34. The photograph shows the end of the ROM in radial deviation. The subject is seated on a low stool so that her humerus is supported on the table when the glenohumeral joint is in 90 degrees of abduction. The examiner's right hand prevents flexion of the subject's elbow beyond 90 degrees when the wrist is moved into radial deviation. The examiner's left hand supports the weight of the subject's hand. The examiner avoids moving the wrist into either flexion or extension.

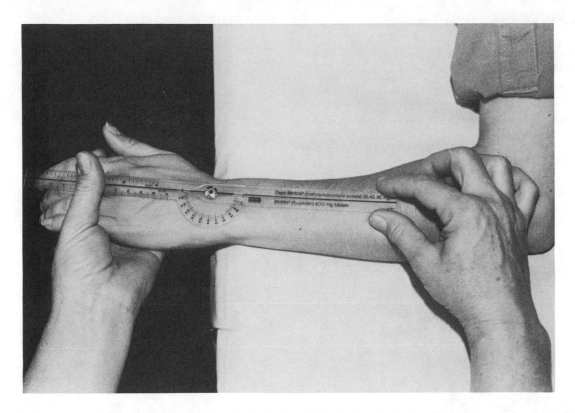

FIGURE 3-35. The starting positions are the same for measuring both radial and ulnar deviation. The goniometer body is centered on the dorsal aspect of the wrist, close to the capitate. The proximal goniometer arm is aligned with the subjects left lateral epicondyle. The distal goniometer arm is aligned along the third metacarpal. The examiner's left hand supports the weight of the subject's hand across the metacarpals and holds the proximal goniometer arm in correct alignment. The examiner keeps the hand in the same plane as the forearm and avoids wrist flexion and extension.

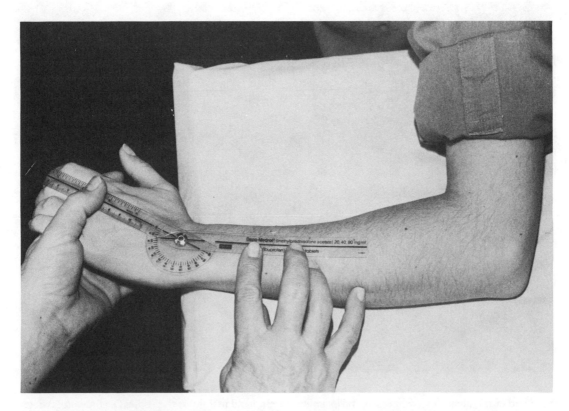

FIGURE 3-36. At the end of the radial deviation ROM, the examiner supports the hand at the level of metacarpals so that the wrist is maintained in a neutral position relative to flexion and extension. The examiner's right hand maintains the goniometer's proximal arm in alignment with the subject's left lateral epicondyle.

ULNAR DEVIATION (Ulnar Flexion)

RECOMMENDED TESTING POSITION AND STABILIZATION (Fig. 3-37)

The testing position is the same as for radial deviation of the wrist.

PHYSIOLOGIC END-FEEL

The end-feel is firm because of tension in the radial collateral ligament and the radial portion of the joint capsule.

GONIOMETER ALIGNMENT (Figs. 3-38 and 3-39)

The alignment is the same as for radial deviation of the wrist.

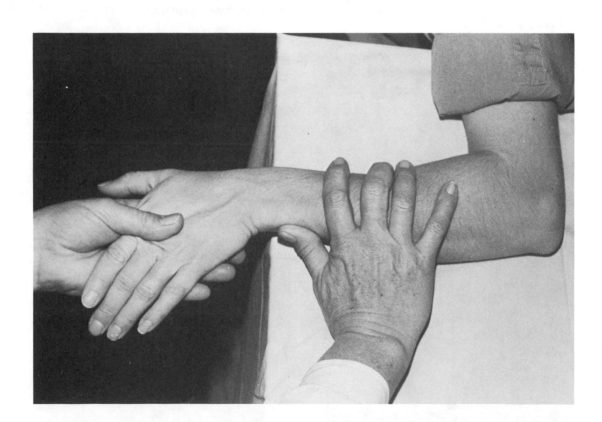

FIGURE 3-37. At the end of the ulnar deviation ROM, the examiner's right hand maintains the subject's elbow in 90 degrees of flexion by preventing elbow extension. The examiner's left hand supports the weight of the subject's hand and maintains the wrist in a neutral position relative to flexion and extension. By firmly grasping the subject's second and third metacarpals, the examiner is able to control motion at the wrist.

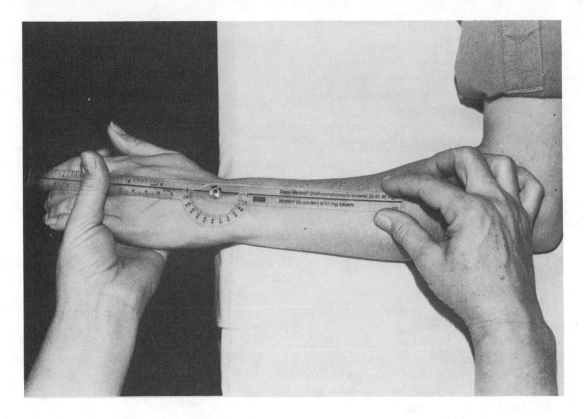

FIGURE 3-38. The starting position for measuring ulnar deviation is the same as the starting position for measuring radial deviation.

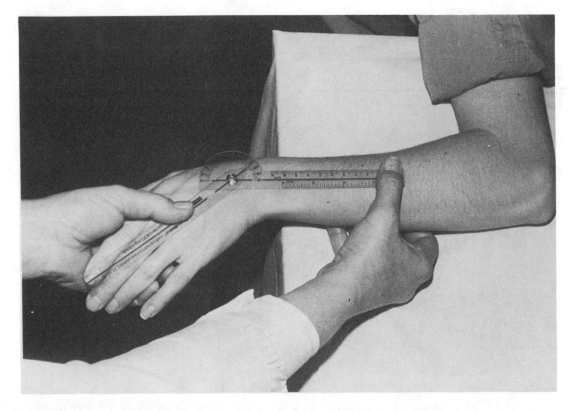

FIGURE 3-39. At the end of the ulnar deviation ROM, the examiner's right hand maintains the proximal goniometer arm in alignment with the lateral epicondyle of the humerus. The examiner's left hand keeps the distal goniometer arm aligned with the subject's third metacarpal.

THE FINGERS

Included in this section are common clinical techniques for measuring motions of the fingers and thumb. These techniques are appropriate for evaluating most people. However, swelling and bony deformities sometimes require the examiner to create alternative evaluation techniques. Photocopies, photographs, and tracings of the hand at the beginning and end of the ROM may be especially helpful.

METACARPOPHALANGEAL (MCP) JOINTS

FLEXION

Motion occurs in the sagittal plane around a coronal axis.

RECOMMENDED TESTING POSITION

Position the subject sitting, with the forearm midway between pronation and supination. The wrist is positioned in 0 degrees of flexion and extension and radial and ulnar deviation. The forearm and hand rest on a supporting surface. The MCP joint being examined should be in a neutral position relative to abduction and adduction. Avoid extreme flexion of the proximal (PIP) and distal (DIP) interphalangeal joints of the finger being examined. (If the wrist and the PIP and DIP joints of the finger being tested are held in flexion, tension in the extensor digitorum communis, extensor indicis, or extensor digiti minimi muscles will restrict the motion.)

STABILIZATION (Fig. 3-40)

Stabilize the metacarpal to prevent wrist motion. Do not hold the MCP joints of the other fingers in extension, as tension in the transverse metacarpal ligament will restrict the motion.

PHYSIOLOGIC END-FEEL

The end-feel may be hard because of contact between the palmar aspect of the proximal phalanx and metacarpal, or the end-feel may be firm because of tension in the dorsal joint capsule and the collateral ligaments.

GONIOMETER ALIGNMENT (Figs. 3-41 and 3-42)

1. Center the fulcrum of the goniometer over the dorsal aspect of the MCP joint.
2. Align the proximal arm over the dorsal midline of the metacarpal.
3. Align the distal arm over the dorsal midline of the proximal phalanx.

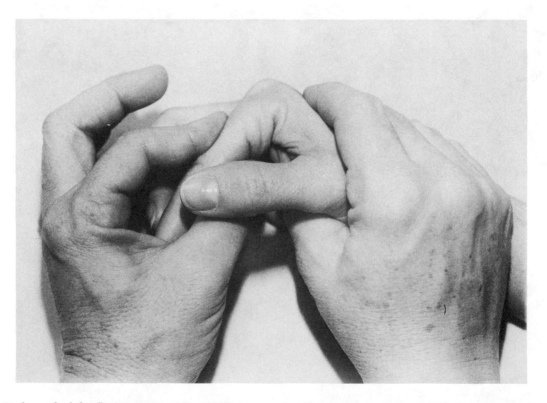

FIGURE 3-40. At the end of the flexion ROM of the subject's second MCP joint, the examiner's right hand is stabilizing the subject's second metacarpal and maintaining the wrist in a neutral position relative to flexion and extension. The examiner's left index finger and thumb grasp the subject's proximal phalanx and maintain the second MCP joint in flexion.

MEASUREMENT OF JOINT MOTION: A GUIDE TO GONIOMETRY

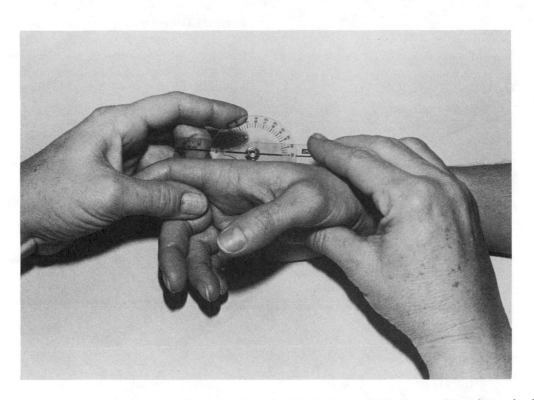

FIGURE 3-41. In the starting position for MCP flexion, the body of the plastic half-circle goniometer is positioned over the dorsal aspect of the subject's second MCP joint. The proximal arm of the goniometer is held on the dorsal midline of the subject's second metacarpal by the examiner's right hand. The distal goniometer arm is aligned on the dorsal midline of the subject's second proximal phalanx. The examiner's left thumb supports the subject's proximal phalanx and helps to maintain the second MCP joint in a neutral position relative to abduction and adduction.

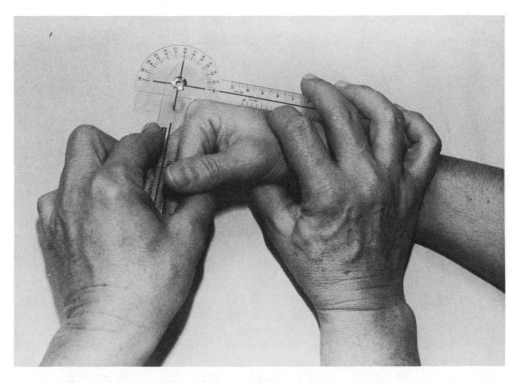

FIGURE 3-42. At the end of MCP flexion, the examiner's right hand holds the proximal goniometer arm in alignment and stabilizes the subject's second metacarpal. Notice that the fulcrum of the goniometer lies somewhat distal and superior to the MCP joint.

UPPER EXTREMITY TESTING

EXTENSION

Motion occurs in the sagittal plane around a coronal axis.

RECOMMENDED TESTING POSITION

Position the subject sitting, with the forearm midway between pronation and supination. The wrist is positioned in 0 degrees of flexion and extension and radial and ulnar deviation. The forearm and hand rest on a supporting surface. The MCP joint being examined should be in a neutral position relative to abduction and adduction. Avoid extension or extreme flexion of the PIP and DIP joints of the finger being tested. (If the PIP and DIP joints are positioned in extension, tension in the flexor digitorum superficialis and profundus muscles may restrict the motion. If the PIP and DIP joints are positioned in full flexion, tension in the lumbricals and interossei will restrict the motion.)

STABILIZATION (Fig. 3-43)

Stabilize the metacarpal to prevent wrist motion. Do not hold the MCP joints of the other fingers in full flexion, as tension in the transverse metacarpal ligament will restrict the motion.

PHYSIOLOGIC END-FEEL

The end-feel is firm because of tension in palmar joint capsule and palmar fibrocartilaginous plate (palmar ligament).

GONIOMETER ALIGNMENT (Figs. 3-44 and 3-45)

The alignment is the same as for flexion of the MCP joint.

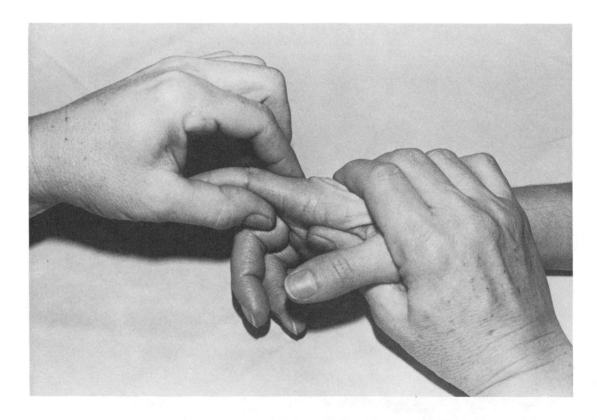

FIGURE 3-43. At the end of MCP extension, the examiner's left index finger and thumb are grasping the subject's second proximal phalanx and maintaining MCP extension. The examiner's right hand maintains the subject's wrist in neutral and stabilizes the second metacarpal.

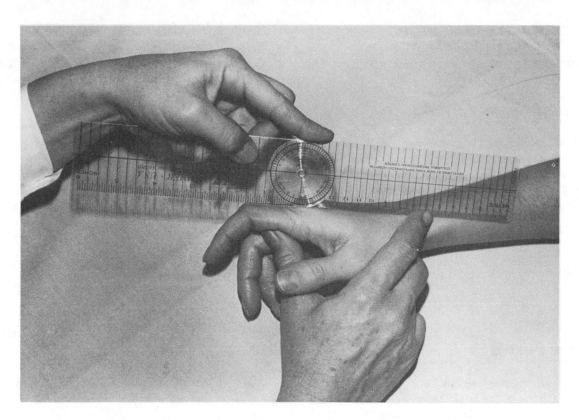

FIGURE 3-44. In the photograph, a full-circle plastic goniometer is being used to measure the extension ROM at the subject's second MCP joint. The proximal arm of the goniometer is slightly longer than it should be for optional alignment. If an appropriate size goniometer is not available, the arms of a plastic goniometer may be cut to a suitable size.

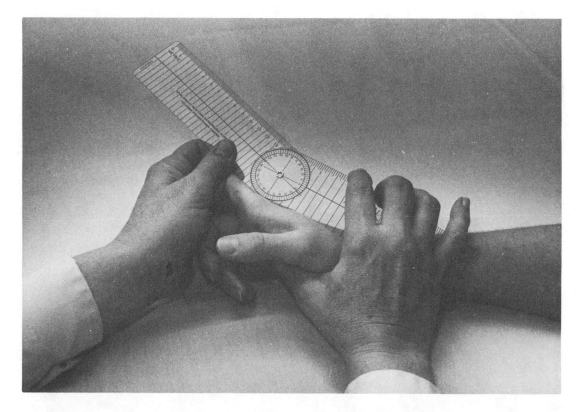

FIGURE 3-45. At the end of MCP extension, the body of the goniometer is aligned over the dorsal aspect of the subject's second MCP joint. The examiner's right hand maintains the subject's wrist in a neutral position and holds the proximal goniometer arm aligned over the subject's second metacarpal. It is easy to see that the subject's ROM in extension is smaller than her ROM in flexion.

ABDUCTION

Motion in the frontal plane around an anterior-posterior axis.

RECOMMENDED TESTING POSITION

Position the subject sitting, with the wrist in 0 degrees of flexion and extension and radial and ulnar deviation. The forearm is fully pronated so that the palm of the hand faces the ground. The MCP joint is in 0 degrees of flexion and extension. The forearm and hand rest on a supporting surface.

STABILIZATION (Fig. 3-46)

Stabilize the metacarpal to prevent wrist motions.

PHYSIOLOGIC END-FEEL

The end-feel is firm because of tension in the collateral ligaments of the MCP joints, the fascia of the web space between the fingers, and the palmar interossei muscles.

GONIOMETER ALIGNMENT (Figs. 3-47 and 3-48)

1. Center the fulcrum of the goniometer over the dorsal aspect of the MCP joint.
2. Align the proximal arm over the dorsal midline of the metacarpal.
3. Align the distal arm over the dorsal midline of the proximal phalanx.

ADDUCTION

Motion occurs in the frontal plane around an anterior-posterior axis.

RECOMMENDED TESTING POSITION, STABILIZATION, AND GONIOMETER ALIGNMENT

The testing position, stabilization, and alignment are the same as for measuring abduction of the MCP joints of the fingers.

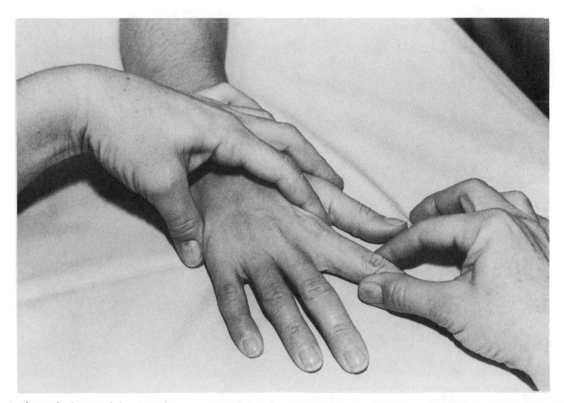

FIGURE 3-46. At the end of MCP abduction, the examiner's left index finger presses against the subject's second metacarpal and prevents radial deviation at the wrist. The examiner's right index finger and thumb are used to maintain the subject's second MCP joint in abduction. The examiner is careful to avoid either lifting up or pressing down on the subject's second proximal phalanx.

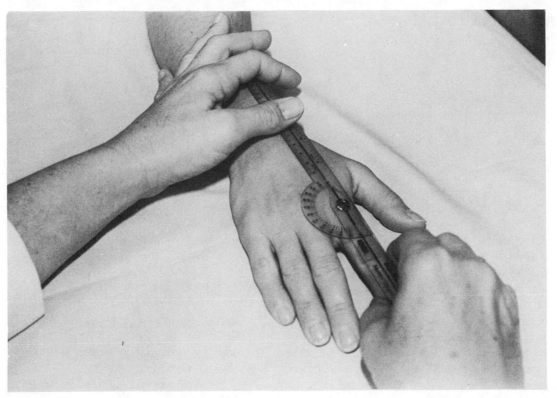

FIGURE 3-47. In the starting position for MCP abduction, the proximal arm of the goniometer is aligned along the dorsal midline of the subject's second metacarpal. The distal goniometer arm is aligned over the dorsal midline of the subject's second proximal phalanx.

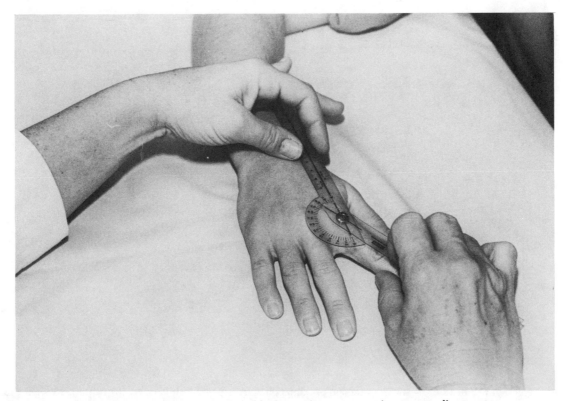

FIGURE 3-48. At the end of MCP abduction, the examiner holds the goniometer arms in correct alignment.

PROXIMAL INTERPHALANGEAL (PIP) JOINT

FLEXION

Motion occurs in the sagittal plane around a coronal axis.

RECOMMENDED TESTING POSITION

Position the subject sitting, with the forearm in 0 degrees of supination and pronation. The wrist is positioned in 0 degrees of flexion and extension and radial and ulnar deviation. The MCP joint is positioned in 0 degrees of flexion, extension, abduction, and adduction. The forearm and hand rest on a supporting surface. (If the wrist and MCP joints are positioned in full flexion, tension in the extensor digitorum communis, extensor indicis, or extensor digiti minimi muscles will restrict the motion. If the MCP joint is positioned in full extension, tension in the lumbricals and interossei muscles will restrict the motion.)

STABILIZATION (Fig. 3-49)

Stabilize the proximal phalanx to prevent motion of the wrist and MCP joint.

PHYSIOLOGIC END-FEEL

Usually the end-feel is hard because of contact between the palmar aspect of the middle phalanx and the proximal phalanx. In some individuals, the end-feel may be soft because of compression of soft tissue between the palmar aspect of the middle and proximal phalanges. In other individuals, the end-feel may be firm because of tension in the dorsal joint capsule and the collateral ligaments.

GONIOMETER ALIGNMENT (Figs. 3-50 and 3-51)

1. Center the fulcrum of the goniometer over the dorsal aspect of the PIP joint.
2. Align the proximal arm over the dorsal midline of the proximal phalanx.
3. Align the distal arm over the dorsal midline of the middle phalanx.

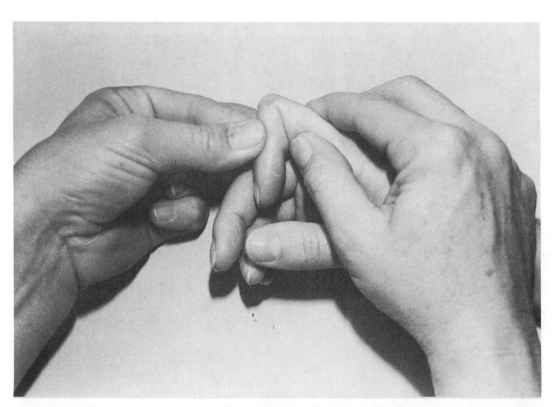

FIGURE 3-49. At the end of PIP flexion the subject's second proximal phalanx is being stabilized by the examiner's right thumb and index finger. The examiner's left thumb and index finger are being used to maintain the subject's PIP joint in full flexion.

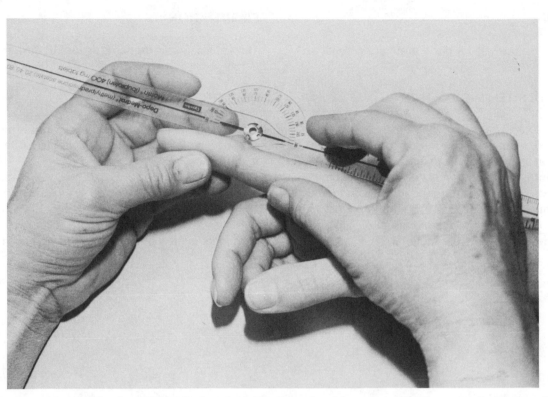

FIGURE 3-50. In the starting position for PIP joint flexion, the subject's hand and forearm rest on the supporting surface. The examiner's right hand holds the proximal arm of the goniometer along the dorsal midline of the subject's second proximal phalanx and maintains the subject's MCP joint in a neutral position relative to flexion and extension. The examiners left thumb supports the subject's middle phalanx.

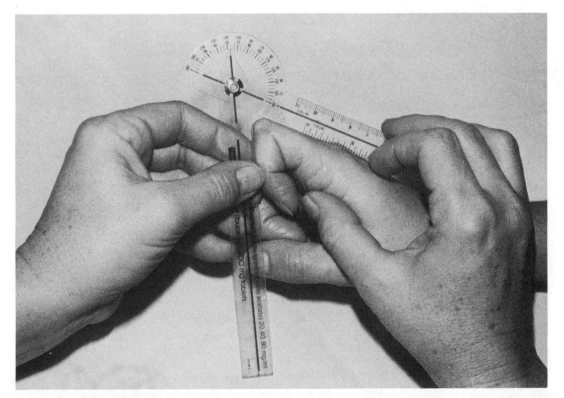

FIGURE 3-51. At the end of PIP flexion, the examiner's right thumb continues to stabilize the subject's MCP joint. The examiner's left thumb is being used to hold the distal goniometer arm in alignment over the dorsal midline of the subject's middle phalanx. The fulcrum of the goniometer lies distal and superior to the PIP joint axis.

EXTENSION

Motion occurs in the sagittal plane around a coronal axis.

RECOMMENDED TESTING POSITION

Position the subject sitting, with the forearm in 0 degrees of supination and pronation. The wrist is positioned in 0 degrees of flexion and extension and radial and ulnar deviation. The MCP joint is positioned in 0 degrees of flexion, extension, abduction, and adduction. The forearm and hand rest on a supporting surface. (If the MCP joint and wrist are extended, tension in the flexor digitorum superficialis and profundus muscles will restrict the motion.)

STABILIZATION

The stabilization is the same as for PIP flexion of the fingers.

PHYSIOLOGIC END-FEEL

The end-feel is firm because of tension in the palmar joint capsule and palmar fibrocartilaginous plate (palmar ligament).

GONIOMETER ALIGNMENT

Alignment is the same as for PIP flexion of the fingers.

DISTAL INTERPHALANGEAL (DIP) JOINT

FLEXION

Motion occurs in the sagittal plane around a coronal axis.

RECOMMENDED TESTING POSITION

Position the subject sitting, with the forearm in 0 degrees of supination and pronation. The wrist is positioned in 0 degrees of flexion and extension and radial and ulnar deviation. The MCP joint is positioned in 0 degrees of flexion, extension, abduction, and adduction. The PIP joint is positioned in approximately 70 to 90 degrees of flexion. The forearm and hand rest on a supporting surface. (If the wrist and MCP and PIP joints are fully flexed, tension in the extensor digitorum communis, extensor indicis, or extensor digiti minimi muscles may restrict the motion. If the PIP joint is extended, tension in the oblique retinacular ligament may restrict the motion even more.)

STABILIZATION

Stabilize the middle phalanx to prevent further flexion or extension of the wrist and MCP and PIP joints.

PHYSIOLOGIC END-FEEL

The end-feel is firm because of tension in the dorsal joint capsule, the collateral ligaments, and the oblique retinacular ligament.

GONIOMETER ALIGNMENT

1. Center the fulcrum of the goniometer over the dorsal aspect of the DIP joint.

2. Align the proximal arm over the dorsal midline of the middle phalanx.
3. Align the distal arm over the dorsal midline of the distal phalanx.

EXTENSION

Motion occurs in the sagittal plane around a coronal axis.

RECOMMENDED TESTING POSITION

Position the subject sitting, with the forearm in 0 degrees of supination and pronation. The wrist is positioned in 0 degrees of flexion and extension and radial and ulnar deviation. The MCP joint is positioned in 0 degrees of flexion, extension, abduction, and adduction. The PIP joint is positioned in approximately 70 to 90 degrees of flexion. The forearm and hand rest on a supporting surface. (If the PIP joint, MCP joint, and wrist are fully extended, tension in the flexor digitorum profundus may restrict the motion.)

STABILIZATION

Stabilize the middle phalanx to prevent extension of the wrist and MCP and PIP joints.

PHYSIOLOGIC END-FEEL

The end-feel is firm because of tension in the palmar joint capsule and the palmar fibrocartilaginous plate (palmar ligament).

GONIOMETER ALIGNMENT

The alignment is the same as for DIP flexion of the fingers.

THE THUMB: CARPOMETACARPAL (CMC) JOINT

FLEXION

Motion occurs in the frontal plane around an anterior-posterior axis, when the subject is in the anatomic position.

RECOMMENDED TESTING POSITION

Position the subject sitting, with the forearm in full supination. The wrist is positioned in 0 degrees of flexion and extension and radial and ulnar deviation. The CMC joint of the thumb is in 0 degrees of abduction and adduction. The MCP and IP joints of the thumb are positioned in 0 degrees of flexion and extension. The forearm and hand rest on a supporting surface. (If the MCP and IP joints of the thumb are positioned in full flexion, tension in the extensor pollicis longus may restrict the motion.)

STABILIZATION (Fig. 3-52)

Stabilize the carpal bones to prevent wrist motions.

PHYSIOLOGIC END-FEEL

The end-feel may be soft because of contact between muscle bulk of the thenar eminence and the palm of the hand; or the end-feel may be firm because of tension in the dorsal joint capsule and the extensor pollicis brevis and abductor pollicis brevis muscles.

GONIOMETER ALIGNMENT (Figs. 3-53 and 3-54)

1. Center the fulcrum of the goniometer over the palmar aspect of the first CMC joint.
2. Align the proximal arm with the palmar midline of the radius.
3. Align the distal arm with the palmar midline of the first metacarpal.

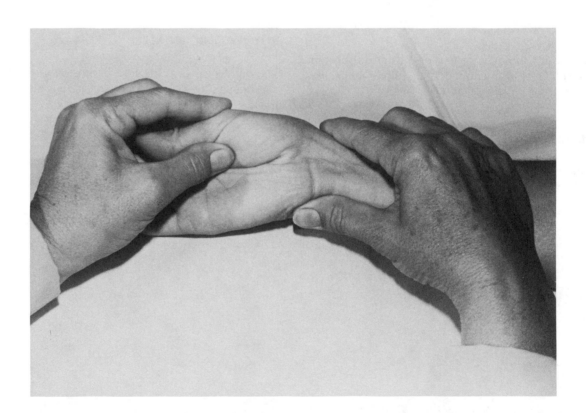

FIGURE 3-52. The subject is shown at the end of the carpometacarpal flexion ROM. The examiner's left hand maintains flexion by pulling medially on the subject's right first metacarpal. The examiner's right hand grasps the subject's carpal bones to prevent both ulnar deviation and palmar flexion.

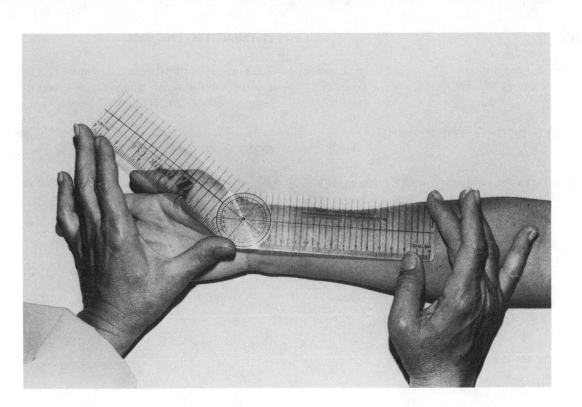

FIGURE 3-53. In the starting position for measuring carpometacarpal flexion, the examiner aligns the proximal goniometer arm so that it is parallel with the radius. The examiner aligns the distal goniometer arm with the subject's first metacarpal.

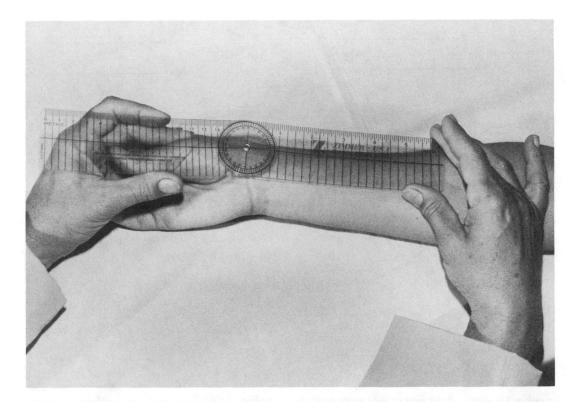

FIGURE 3-54. At the end of the flexion ROM the examiner's left hand maintains both flexion and alignment of the distal goniometer arm. The examiner's right hand keeps the proximal goniometer arm parallel to the radius.

EXTENSION

Motion occurs in the frontal plane around an anterior-posterior axis, when the subject is in anatomic position.

RECOMMENDED TESTING POSITION AND STABILIZATION (Fig. 3-55)

The testing position and stabilization are the same as for flexion of the CMC joint of the thumb.

PHYSIOLOGIC END-FEEL

The end-feel is firm because of tension in the anterior joint capsule and the flexor pollicis brevis, adductor pollicis, opponens pollicis, and first dorsal interossei muscles.

GONIOMETER ALIGNMENT (Figs. 3-56 and 3-57)

The alignment is the same as for flexion of the CMC joint of the thumb.

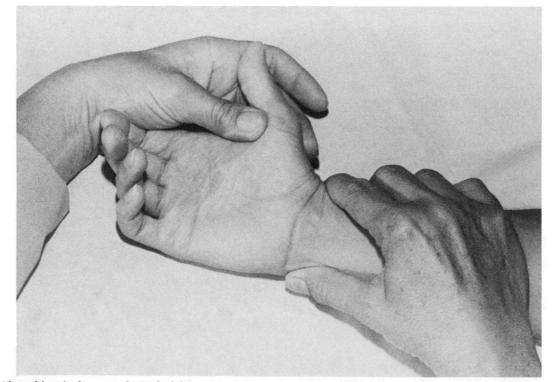

FIGURE 3-55. The subject is shown at the end of the carpometacarpal extension ROM. The examiner uses her left thumb and third finger to pull the metacarpal laterally into extension. The examiner places her right hand on the subject's carpal bones to prevent both radial deviation and palmar flexion.

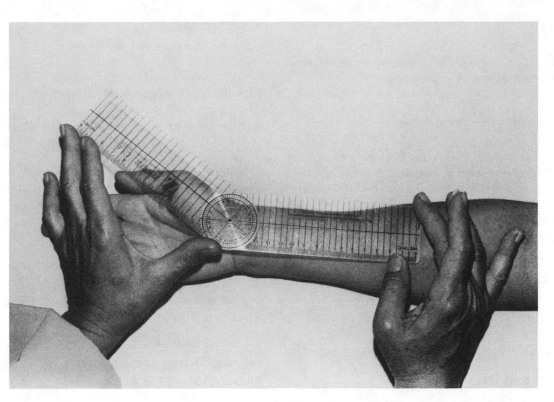

FIGURE 3-56. In the starting position for measuring carpometacarpal extension, goniometer alignment is the same as for measuring carpometacarpal flexion.

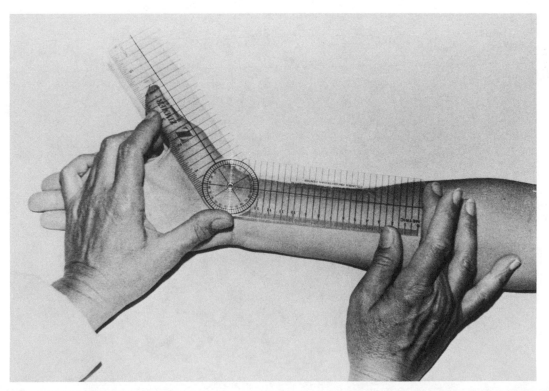

FIGURE 3-57. At the end of carpometacarpal extension the examiner's left hand keeps the distal goniometer arm aligned with the first metacarpal and also holds the thumb in extension. The examiner's right hand keeps the proximal goniometer arm aligned with the subject's radius.

ABDUCTION

Motion occurs in the sagittal plane around a coronal axis, when the subject is in anatomic position.

RECOMMENDED TESTING POSITION

Position the subject sitting, with the forearm midway between supination and pronation. The wrist is positioned in 0 degrees of flexion and extension and radial and ulnar deviation. The CMC, MCP, and IP joints of the thumb are positioned in 0 degrees of flexion and extension. The forearm and hand rest on a supporting surface.

STABILIZATION (Fig. 3-58)

Stabilize the carpal bones and the second metacarpal to prevent wrist motions.

PHYSIOLOGIC END-FEEL

The end-feel is firm because of tension in the fascia and skin of the web space between the thumb and index finger. Tension in the adductor pollicis and first dorsal interossei muscles also contribute to the firm end-feel.

GONIOMETER ALIGNMENT (Figs. 3-59 and 3-60)

1. Center the fulcrum of the goniometer midway between the dorsal aspect of the first and second carpometacarpal joints.
2. Align the proximal arm with the lateral midline of the second metacarpal.
3. Align the distal arm with the lateral midline of the first metacarpal.

ADDUCTION

Motion occurs in the sagittal plane around a coronal axis, when the subject is in anatomic position.

RECOMMENDED TESTING POSITION, STABILIZATION, AND GONIOMETER ALIGNMENT

The testing position, stabilization, and alignment are the same as for abduction of the CMC joint of the thumb.

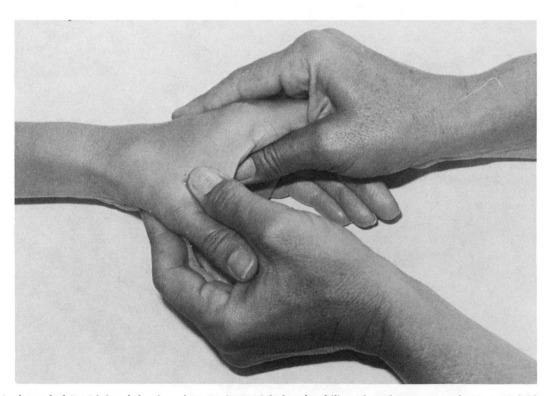

FIGURE 3-58. At the end of CMC joint abduction, the examiner's right hand stabilizes the subject's second metacarpal. The examiner's left thumb and index finger are grasping the subject's first metacarpal and maintaining abduction. The first metacarpal is grasped just proximal to the MCP joint.

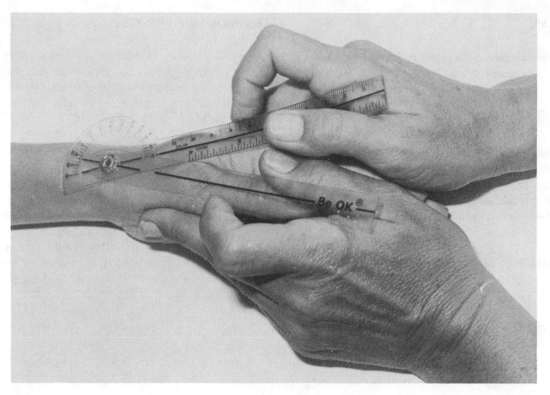

FIGURE 3-59. In the starting position for CMC abduction, the subject's first and second metacarpals are separated slightly; therefore, when the arms of the goniometer are aligned with the first and second metacarpals, the goniometer will not be at 0 degrees.

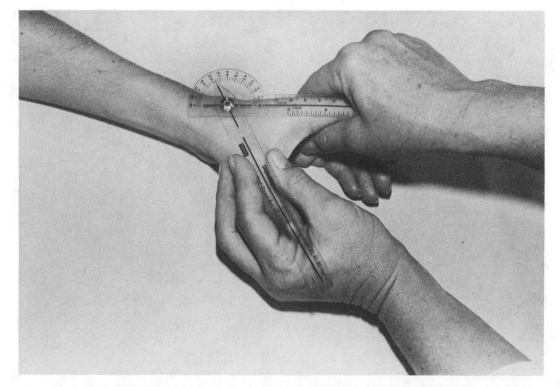

FIGURE 3-60. At the end of CMC abduction, the examiner's right hand aligns the proximal goniometer arm with the subject's second metacarpal and at the same time provides stabilization. The examiner's left hand, which is maintaining the alignment of the distal goniometer arm, also maintains abduction.

OPPOSITION

Motion is a combination of flexion, abduction, and medial-axial rotation (pronation).

RECOMMENDED TESTING POSITION

Position the subject sitting, with the forearm in full supination. The wrist is in 0 degrees of flexion and extension and radial and ulnar deviation. The IP joints of the thumb and little finger are positioned in 0 degrees of flexion and extension. The forearm and hand rest on a supporting surface.

STABILIZATION (Fig. 3-61)

Stabilize the fifth metacarpal to prevent wrist motions.

PHYSIOLOGIC END-FEEL

The end-feel may be soft because of contact between the muscle bulk of the thenar eminence and the palm; or the end-feel may be firm because of tension in the joint capsule, extensor pollicis brevis muscle, and transverse metacarpal ligament (affecting the fifth finger).

GONIOMETER ALIGNMENT (Figs. 3-62 and 3-63)

The goniometer is not commonly used to measure the range of opposition. Instead, a ruler often is used to measure the distance between the tip of the thumb and the tip of the fifth digit. Alternatively, a ruler may be used to measure the distance between the tip of the thumb and the base (MCP Joint) of the fifth finger.

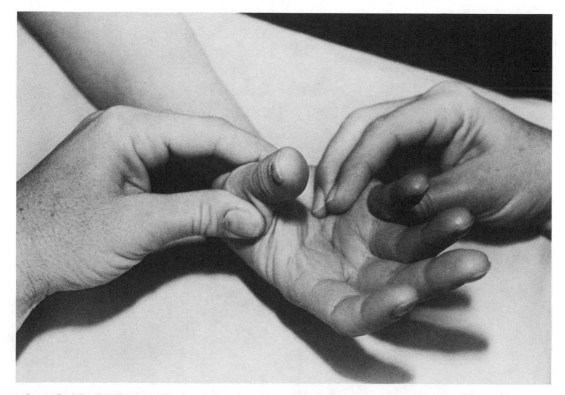

FIGURE 3-61. At the end of the ROM in opposition, the examiner's left hand grasps the subject's thumb at the level of the MCP joint. The examiner is able to maintain the thumb in opposition by exerting pressure on the first metacarpal with her left thumb. The examiner's right hand maintains the fifth metacarpal and proximal phalanx in opposition.

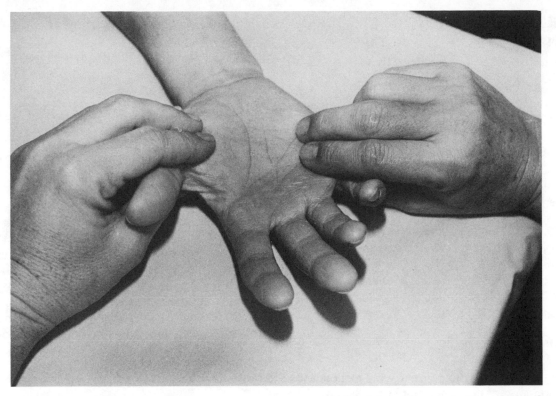

FIGURE 3-62. In the starting position for opposition, the examiner grasps the fifth and first metacarpals. The subject's hand is supported by the table.

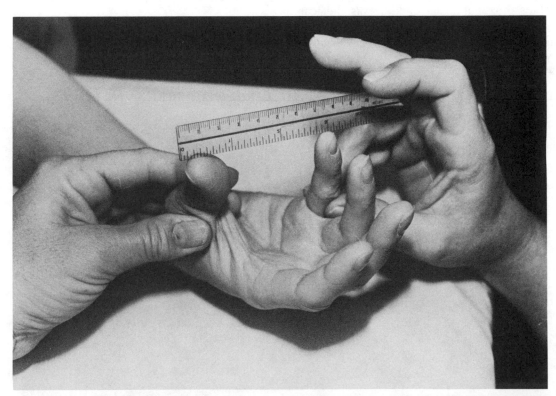

FIGURE 3-63. The ROM in opposition is determined by measuring the distance between the lateral tip of the subject's thumb and the lateral tip of the subject's fifth digit. The examiner is using an arm of a half-circle plastic goniometer as the measuring device; however, any ruler or tape measure would be suitable. The photograph does not show the complete ROM of opposition, because we wished to demonstrate clearly how the ROM is measured. The tip of the subject's fifth finger and the tip of her thumb are touching when the ROM in opposition is completed.

METACARPOPHALANGEAL (MCP) JOINT

FLEXION

Motion occurs in the frontal plane around an anterior-posterior axis, when the subject is in anatomic position.

RECOMMENDED TESTING POSITION

Position the subject sitting, with the forearm in full supination. The wrist is in 0 degrees of flexion and extension and radial and ulnar deviation. The CMC joint of the thumb is positioned in 0 degrees of flexion, extension, abduction, adduction, and opposition. The IP joint of the thumb is in 0 degrees of flexion and extension. The forearm and hand rest on a supporting surface. (If the wrist and IP joint of the thumb are positioned in full flexion, tension in the extensor pollicis longus muscle will restrict the motion.)

STABILIZATION (Fig. 3-64)

Stabilize the first metacarpal to prevent wrist motion and flexion and opposition of the CMC joint of the thumb.

PHYSIOLOGIC END-FEEL

The end-feel may be hard because of contact between the palmar aspect of the proximal phalanx and the first metacarpal; or the end-feel may be firm because of tension in the dorsal joint capsule, the collateral ligaments, and extensor pollicis brevis muscle.

GONIOMETER ALIGNMENT (Figs. 3-65 and 3-66)

1. Center the fulcrum of the goniometer over the dorsal aspect of the MCP joint.

2. Align the proximal arm over the dorsal midline of the metacarpal.
3. Align the distal arm with the dorsal midline of the proximal phalanx.

EXTENSION

Motion occurs in the frontal plane around an anterior-posterior axis, when the subject is in anatomic position.

RECOMMENDED TESTING POSITION

Position the subject sitting, with the forearm in full supination. The wrist is in 0 degrees of flexion and extension and radial and ulnar deviation. The CMC joint of the thumb is positioned in 0 degrees of flexion, extension, abduction, adduction, and opposition. The IP joint of the thumb is in 0 degrees of flexion and extension. The forearm and hand rest on a supporting surface. (If the IP joint of the thumb is positioned in full extension, tension in the flexor pollicis longus may restrict the motion.)

STABILIZATION

Stabilize the first metacarpal to prevent motion at the wrist and CMC joint of the thumb.

PHYSIOLOGIC END-FEEL

The end-feel is firm because of tension in the palmar joint capsule, palmar fibrocartilaginous plate (palmar ligament), intersesamoid ligament, and the flexor pollicis brevis muscle.

GONIOMETER ALIGNMENT

The alignment is the same as for flexion of the MCP joint of the thumb.

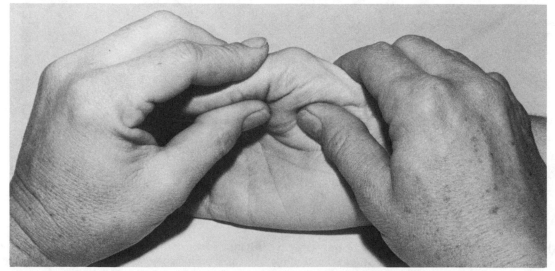

FIGURE 3-64. At the end of MCP joint flexion, the examiner's right thumb and index finger stabilize the subject's first metacarpal. The examiner's left index finger maintains the subject's MCP joint in flexion through pressure on the subject's proximal phalanx. The examiner's left thumb helps to prevent flexion at the subject's IP joint.

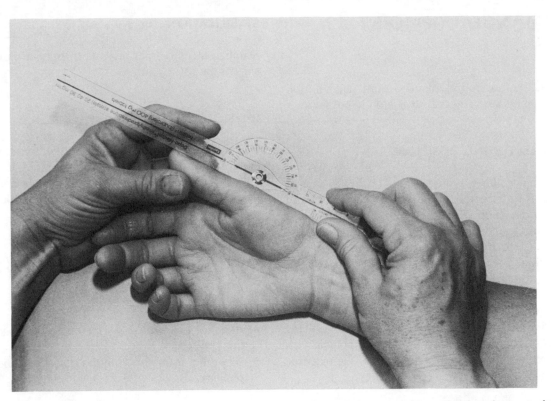

FIGURE 3-65. In the starting position for MCP flexion, the fulcrum of the goniometer is centered over the dorsal aspect of the MCP joint. The distal goniometer arm is aligned along the dorsal midline of the proximal phalanx. The examiner's left hand holds the distal goniometer arm in alignment and maintains the IP joint in extension. The proximal goniometer is aligned along the dorsal midline of the subject's first metacarpal.

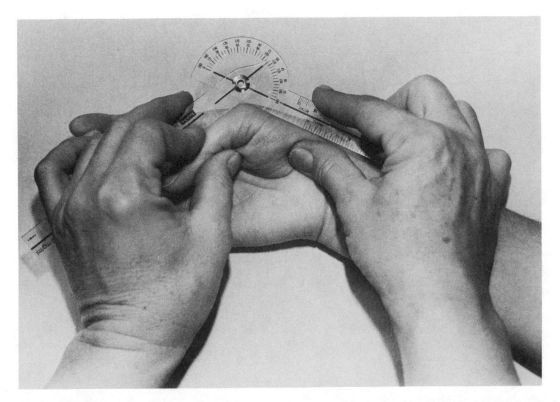

FIGURE 3-66. At the end of MCP flexion, the examiner's left hand stabilizes the subject's IP joint and maintains alignment of the distal arm of the goniometer. The examiner uses her right hand to stabilize the subject's first metacarpal and to keep the proximal arm of the goniometer in correct alignment.

UPPER EXTREMITY TESTING

INTERPHALANGEAL (IP) JOINT

FLEXION

Motion occurs in the frontal plane around an anterior-posterior axis, when the subject is in anatomic position.

RECOMMENDED TESTING POSITION

Position the subject sitting, with the forearm in full supination. The wrist is in 0 degrees of flexion and extension and radial and ulnar deviation. The CMC joint is positioned in 0 degrees of flexion, extension, abduction, adduction, and opposition. The MCP joint of the thumb is in 0 degrees of flexion and extension. The forearm and hand rest on a supporting surface. (If the wrist and MCP joint of the thumb are flexed, tension in the extensor pollicis longus may restrict the motion. If the MCP joint of the thumb is fully extended, tension in the first palmar interossei, the abductor pollicis brevis, and the oblique fibers of the adductor pollicis may restrict the motion through their insertion into the extensor hood mechanism.)

STABILIZATION (Fig. 3-67)

Stabilize the proximal phalanx to prevent flexion or extension of the MCP joint.

PHYSIOLOGIC END-FEEL

Usually, the end-feel is firm because of tension in the collateral ligaments and the dorsal joint capsule. In some individuals, the end-feel may be hard because of contact between the palmar aspect of the distal phalanx, the fibrocartilaginous plate, and the proximal phalanx.

GONIOMETER ALIGNMENT (Figs. 3-68 and 3-69)

1. Center the fulcrum of the goniometer over the dorsal surface of the IP joint.
2. Align the proximal arm with the dorsal aspect of the proximal phalanx.
3. Align the distal arm with the dorsal midline of the distal phalanx.

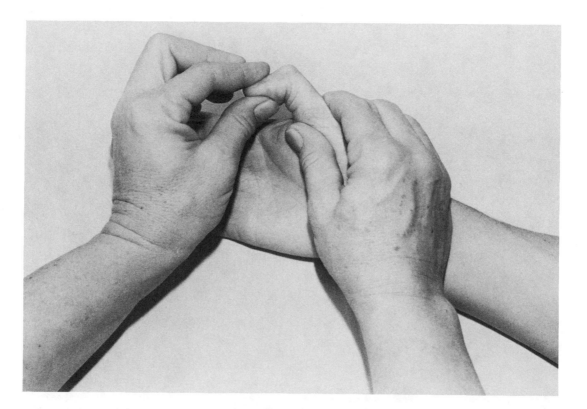

FIGURE 3-67. At the end of the ROM of IP flexion, the examiner's right thumb and index finger are being used to maintain the subject's MCP joint in 0 degrees of flexion. The examiner's right hand also keeps the subject's CMC joint in 0 degrees of abduction and opposition. The examiner's left thumb and index finger are used to maintain the subject's IP joint in flexion.

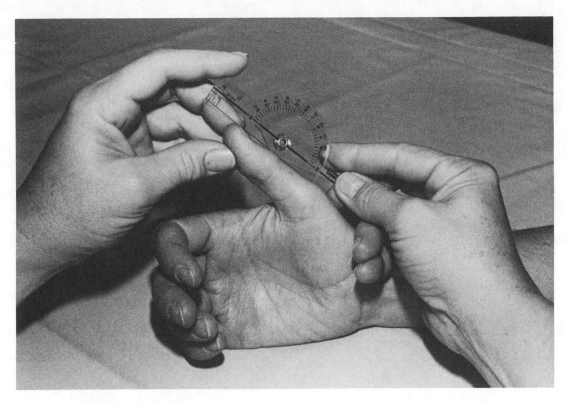

FIGURE 3-68. The examiner is using a plastic half-circle goniometer with the arms cut off. The proximal goniometer arm is aligned on the dorsal midline of the subject's first proximal phalanx. The distal goniometer arm is aligned along the subject's first distal phalanx.

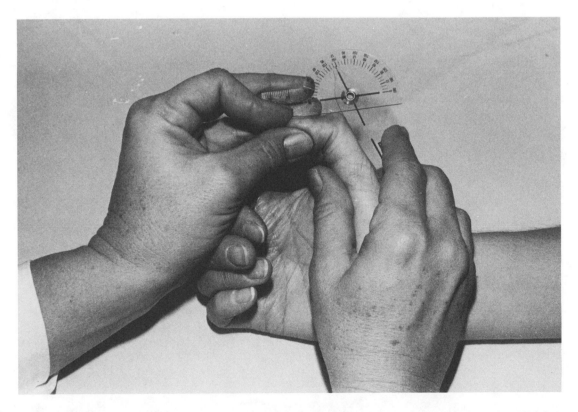

FIGURE 3-69. At the end of the flexion ROM, the examiner's right hand stabilizes the subject's CMC and MCP joints and holds the shortened proximal goniometer arm in alignment. The examiner's left hand holds the distal goniometer arm in alignment and maintains the IP joint in flexion through pressure on the subject's distal phalanx. The fulcrum of the goniometer lies distal and superior to the IP joint.

UPPER EXTREMITY TESTING

EXTENSION

Motion occurs in the frontal plane around an anterior-posterior axis, when the subject is in anatomic position.

RECOMMENDED TESTING POSITION

Position the subject sitting, with the forearm in full supination. The wrist is in 0 degrees of flexion and extension and radial and ulnar deviation. The CMC joint of the thumb is positioned in 0 degrees of flexion, extension, abduction, adduction, and opposition. The MCP joint of the thumb is in 0 degrees of flexion and extension. The forearm and hand rest on a supporting surface. (If the wrist and MCP joint of the thumb are extended, tension in the flexor pollicis longus may restrict the motion.)

STABILIZATION

The stabilization is the same as for flexion of the IP joint of the thumb.

PHYSIOLOGIC END-FEEL

The end-feel is firm because of tension in the palmar joint capsule and the palmar fibrocartilaginous plate (palmar ligament).

GONIOMETER ALIGNMENT

The alignment is the same as for flexion of the IP joint of the thumb.

LOWER EXTREMITY TESTING

OBJECTIVES

Upon completion of this chapter the reader will be able to:

1. Identify:
   the appropriate planes and axes for each lower extremity joint motion
   the structures that limit the end of the ROM at each lower extremity joint and the expected normal end-feel

2. Describe:
   the recommended testing positions used for each lower extremity

3. List the upper and lower extremity joint motions that can be tested in each of the following positions: supine, prone, and sitting

4. Perform a goniometric evaluation of any lower extremity joint including:
   a clear explanation of the testing procedure
   positioning of the subject in recommended testing position
   adequate stabilization of the proximal joint component
   a correct determination of the end of the ROM
   a correct identification of the end-feel
   palpation of the correct bony landmarks
   accurate alignment of the goniometer
   correct reading and recording

5. Assess the intratester and intertester reliability of goniometric evaluations of the lower extremity joints.

THE HIP: ILIOFEMORAL JOINT

FLEXION

Motion occurs in the sagittal plane around a coronal axis.

RECOMMENDED TESTING POSITION

Position the subject supine with the hip in 0 degrees of abduction, adduction, and rotation. Initially, the knee is extended, but as the range of hip flexion is completed, the knee is allowed to flex. If the knee is kept in extension, tension in the hamstring muscles will restrict the motion.

STABILIZATION (Fig. 4-1) *pelvis*

Stabilize the pelvis to prevent rotation or posterior tilting.

PHYSIOLOGIC END-FEEL *SOFT*

The end-feel is usually soft because of contact between the muscle bulk of the anterior thigh and the lower abdomen.

GONIOMETER ALIGNMENT (Figs. 4-2 and 4-3)

1. Center the fulcrum of the goniometer over the lateral aspect of the hip joint using the greater trochanter of the femur for reference.
2. Align the proximal arm with the lateral midline of the pelvis.
3. Align the distal arm with the lateral midline of the femur using the lateral epicondyle for reference.

normal range = 0-120°

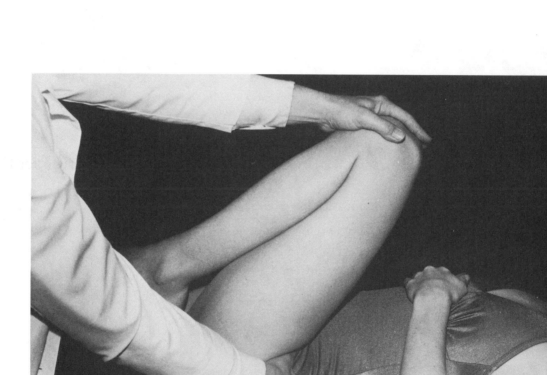

FIGURE 4-1. The subject's left lower extremity is shown at the end of the ROM in hip flexion. The examiner's left hand holds the hip in flexion by pushing on the distal femur. Stress on the knee joint is avoided and the subject's knee is allowed to flex passively. The end of the ROM occurs when motion of the femur causes posterior tilting of the pelvis. Because the examiner's hand is positioned on the pelvis, she is able to detect any pelvic motion.

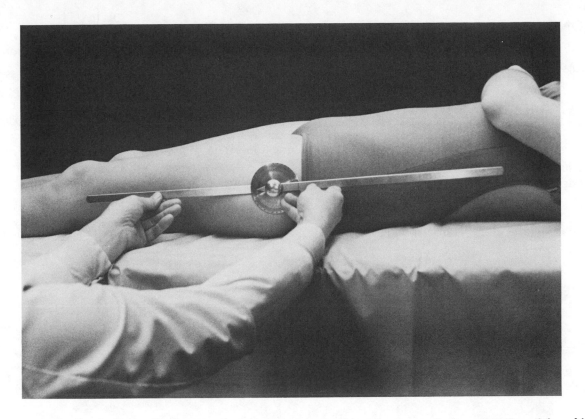

FIGURE 4-2. At the beginning of the ROM, the proximal arm of the goniometer is aligned along the lateral midline of the subject's pelvis. The fulcrum is centered over the subject's greater trochanter, and the distal arm is aligned with the subject's lateral femoral epicondyle.

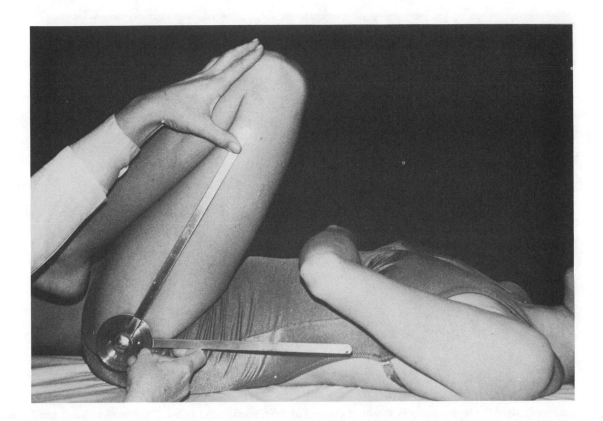

FIGURE 4-3. At the end of the hip flexion ROM, the examiner's left hand holds the distal goniometer arm in alignment and maintains the hip in flexion. The examiner's right hand holds the proximal goniometer arm aligned with the lateral midline of the subject's pelvis.

EXTENSION

Motion occurs in a sagittal plane around a coronal axis.

RECOMMENDED TESTING POSITION

Position the subject prone with the hip in 0 degrees of abduction, adduction, and rotation. The knee is extended. If the knee is flexed, tension in the rectus femoris muscle will restrict the motion. A pillow may be placed under the abdomen for comfort, but no pillow is placed under the head.

STABILIZATION (Fig. 4-4) *Pelvis*

Stabilize the pelvis to prevent rotation or anterior tilting.

PHYSIOLOGIC END-FEEL *Firm*

The end-feel is firm because of tension in the anterior joint capsule, iliofemoral ligament, and, to a lesser extent, the ischiofemoral and pubofemoral ligaments. On occasion, tension in various muscles that flex the hip, such as the iliopsoas, sartorius, tensor fasciae latae, gracilis, and adductor longus, may contribute to the firm end-feel.

GONIOMETER ALIGNMENT (Figs. 4-5 and 4-6)

The alignment is the same as for measuring hip flexion.

Norm = 0-30°

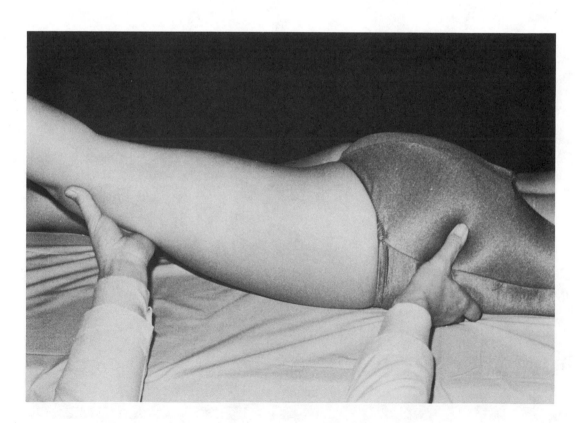

FIGURE 4-4. The subject's right lower extremity is shown at the end of the hip extension ROM. The examiner's left hand supports the distal femur and maintains the hip in extension. The examiner's right hand grasps the subject's pelvis at the level of the anterior superior iliac spine. The end of the ROM occurs when movement of the femur produces anterior tilting of the pelvis. Because the examiner's right hand is on the subject's pelvis, the examiner is able to detect pelvic tilting.

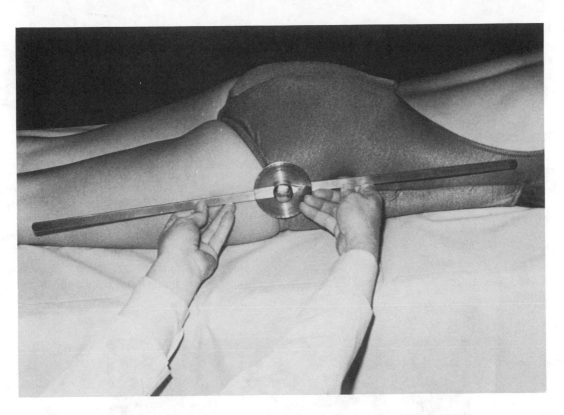

FIGURE 4-5. In the prone starting position, the proximal goniometer arm is aligned with the lateral midline of the subject's pelvis. The distal goniometer arm is aligned along the lateral midline of the subject's thigh, using the lateral femoral epicondyle as a landmark. The fulcrum is aligned over the greater trochanter.

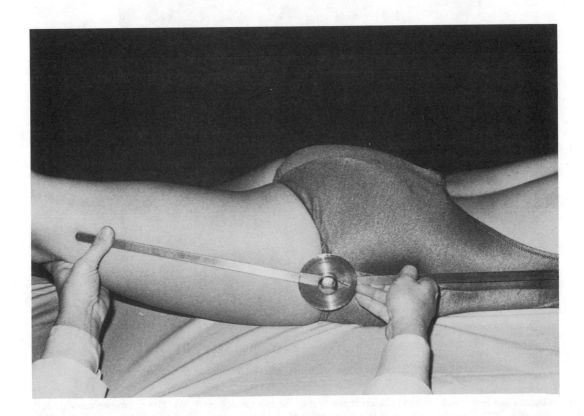

FIGURE 4-6. At the end of the hip extension ROM, the examiner's right hand holds the proximal goniometer arm in correct alignment. The examiner's left hand supports the subject's femur and keeps the distal goniometer arm aligned.

ABDUCTION

Motion occurs in a frontal plane around an anterior-posterior axis.

RECOMMENDED TESTING POSITION

Position the subject supine with the hip in 0 degrees of flexion, extension, and rotation. The knee is extended.

STABILIZATION (Fig. 4-7)

Stabilize the pelvis to prevent rotation and lateral tilting.

Norm 0-45°

PHYSIOLOGIC END-FEEL FIRM

The end-feel is firm because of tension in the inferior (medial) joint capsule, pubofemoral ligament, ischiofemoral ligament, and inferior band of the iliofemoral ligament. Tension in the adductor magnus, adductor longus, adductor brevis, pectineus, and gracilis muscles may contribute to the firm end-feel.

GONIOMETER ALIGNMENT (Figs. 4-8 and 4-9)

1. Center the fulcrum of the goniometer over the anterior superior iliac spine (ASIS) of the extremity being measured.
2. Align the proximal arm with an imaginary horizontal line extending from one ASIS to the other ASIS.
3. Align the distal arm with the anterior midline of the femur using the midline of the patella for reference.

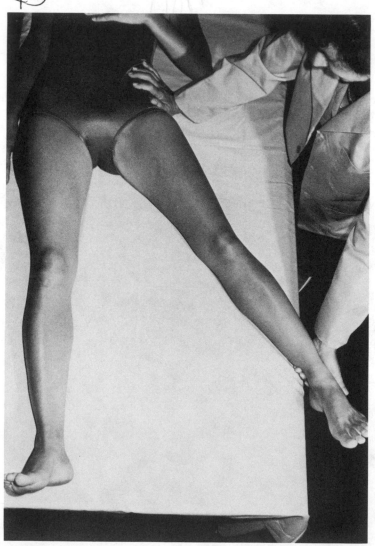

FIGURE 4-7. The subject's left lower extremity is shown at the end of the hip abduction ROM. The examiner uses her left hand to pull the subject's leg into abduction. The examiner's grip on the subject's ankle is designed to prevent lateral rotation of the hip. The end of the ROM occurs when lateral motion of the extremity causes lateral tilting of the pelvis and lateral spinal flexion. The pelvic motion is detected by the examiner's right hand.

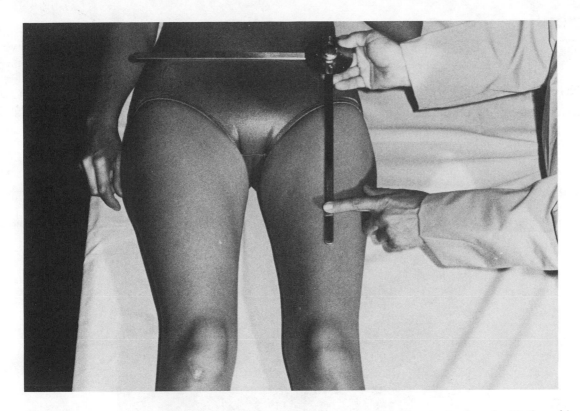

FIGURE 4-8. In the starting position for measuring hip abduction, the proximal goniometer arm is aligned with the subject's anterior superior iliac spines. The distal arm is aligned with the midline of the patella. Although the goniometer is at 90 degrees, this is the 0 starting position. Therefore, the examiner must transpose her reading from 90 degrees to 0 degrees. Example, actual reading: 90–120°; recorded as: 0–30°.

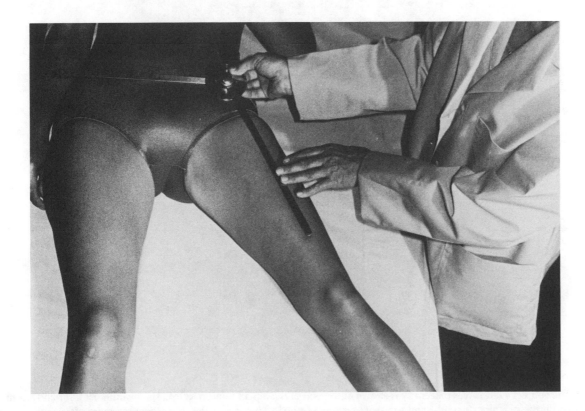

FIGURE 4-9. At the end of the hip abduction ROM, the distal goniometer arm is aligned with the mid-patella, while the proximal arm is aligned with the subject's anterior superior iliac spines.

ADDUCTION

Motion occurs in a frontal plane around an anterior-posterior axis.

RECOMMENDED TESTING POSITION

The testing position is similar to the position used for measuring hip abduction. However, the contralateral hip is abducted to allow the hip being measured to complete its full range of adduction.

STABILIZATION (Fig. 4-10)

Stabilization is the same as for measuring hip abduction.

PHYSIOLOGIC END-FEEL

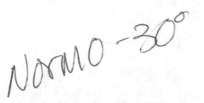

The end-feel is firm because of tension in the superior (lateral) joint capsule and the superior band of the iliofemoral ligament. Tension in the gluteus medius and minimus and the tensor fasciae latae muscles may also contribute to the firm end-feel.

GONIOMETER ALIGNMENT (Figs. 4-11 and 4-12)

The alignment is the same as for measuring hip abduction.

Normo - 30°

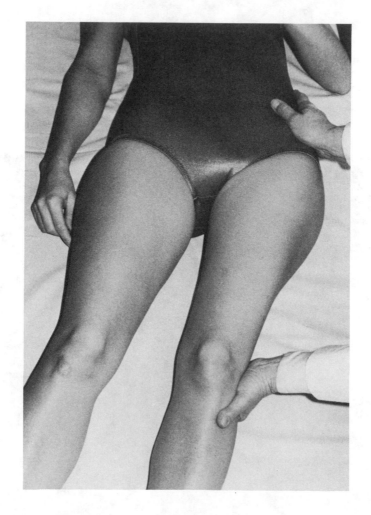

FIGURE 4-10. The subject's left lower extremity is shown at the end of the hip adduction ROM. The examiner's left hand maintains the hip in adduction, while the examiner's right hand grasps the subject's pelvis. The end of the ROM occurs when additional adduction of the extremity causes the subject's pelvis to tilt laterally. Because the examiner's right hand is on the subject's pelvis, the examiner is able to detect any lateral pelvic tilting.

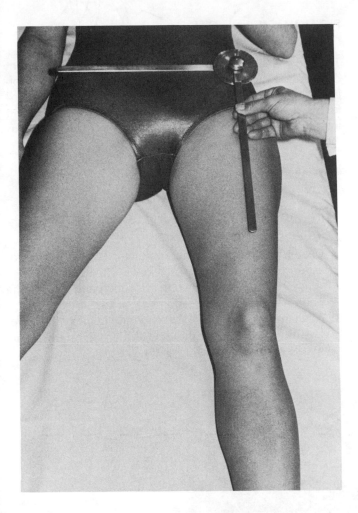

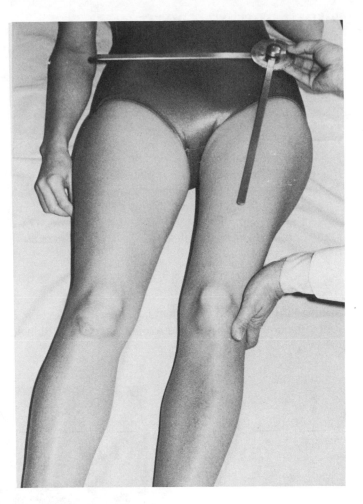

FIGURE 4-11. In the starting position for measuring left hip adduction, the subject's right lower extremity has been abducted to allow adequate space for adduction of the left lower extremity. The proximal goniometer arm is aligned with the subject's anterior superior iliac spines. The distal goniometer arm is aligned along the anterior midline of the subject's femur. This alignment places the goniometer at 90 degrees. Therefore, when the examiner records her measurement, she will transpose the reading so that 90 degrees is equivalent to 0 degrees. Example: actual reading: 90–60°; recorded as: 0–30°.

FIGURE 4-12. At the end of the hip adduction ROM, the examiner's right hand holds the goniometer body over the subject's anterior superior iliac spine. The examiner is able to prevent hip rotation by maintaining a firm grasp at the subject's knee.

MEDIAL (INTERNAL) ROTATION

Motion occurs in a transverse plane around a longitudinal axis, when the subject is in anatomic position.

RECOMMENDED TESTING POSITION

Position the subject sitting on a supporting surface, with the knees flexed to 90 degrees over the edge of the surface. The hip is in 0 degrees of abduction and adduction and in 90 degrees of flexion. A towel roll is placed under the distal end of the femur to maintain the femur in a horizontal plane.

As an alternative, measurements may be taken with the subject either supine or prone. The hip is in 0 degrees of abduction, adduction, and flexion. The knee is flexed to 90 degrees.

STABILIZATION (Fig. 4-13)

Stabilize the distal end of the femur to prevent adduction, or further flexion of the hip. Avoid rotations and lateral tilting of the pelvis.

PHYSIOLOGIC END-FEEL *FIRM*

The end-feel is firm because of tension in the posterior joint capsule and the ischiofemoral ligament. Tension in the following muscles may also contribute to the firm end-feel: piriformis, obturator internus and externus, gemelli superior and inferior, quadratus femoris, the posterior fibers of the gluteus medius and gluteus maximus.

GONIOMETER ALIGNMENT (Figs. 4-14 and 4-15)

1. Center the fulcrum of the goniometer over the anterior aspect of the patella.
2. Align the proximal arm so that it is perpendicular to the floor or parallel to the supporting surface.
3. Align the distal arm with the anterior midline of the lower leg, using the crest of the tibia and a point midway between the two malleoli for reference.

0-45

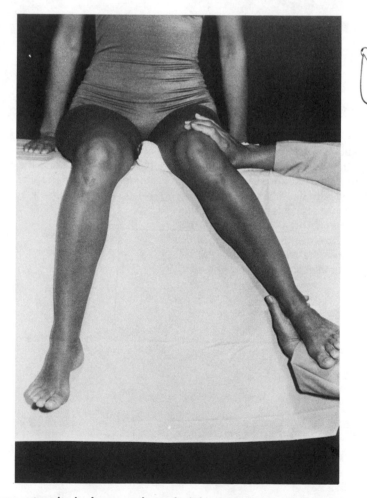

FIGURE 4-13. The subject's left lower extremity is shown at the end of the ROM of hip medial rotation. The examiner's right hand is placed on the subject's distal femur to prevent hip flexion and adduction. The examiner uses her left hand to maintain medial rotation. The subject assists in stabilization by placing both of her hands on the supporting surface and by shifting her weight over her left hip. The examiner watches for any lateral trunk flexion during the motion. When motion of the leg produces lateral flexion of the spine, the end of the ROM has been reached.

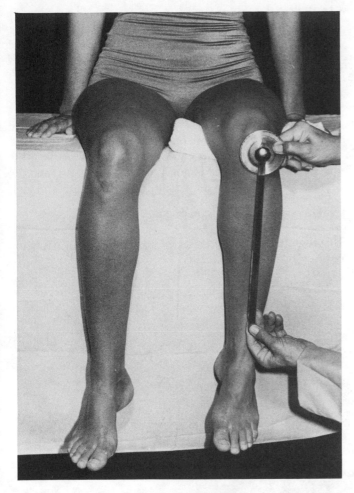

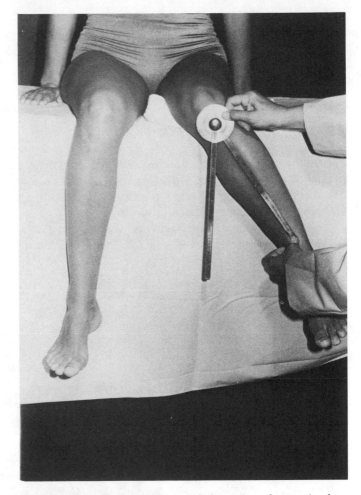

FIGURE 4-14. In the starting position for measuring hip rotation, the fulcrum of the goniometer is placed over the patella. Both arms of the goniometer are together.

FIGURE 4-15. At the end of hip medial rotation, the proximal goniometer arm hangs freely so that it is perpendicular to the floor. The distal goniometer arm is aligned along the crest of the tibia.

LATERAL (EXTERNAL) ROTATION

Motion occurs in a transverse plane around a longitudinal axis, when the subject is in anatomic position.

RECOMMENDED TESTING POSITION

The testing position is similar to the position used to measure medial rotation of the hip. However, the contralateral knee may need to be flexed to allow the hip being measured to complete its full range of lateral rotation.

As an alternative, measurements may be taken with the subject either supine or prone, similar to the position used to measure medial rotation of the hip.

STABILIZATION (Fig. 4-16)

Stabilize the distal end of the femur to prevent abduction or further flexion of the hip. Avoid rotations and lateral tilting of the pelvis.

PHYSIOLOGIC END-FEEL

The end-feel is firm because of tension in the anterior joint capsule, iliofemoral ligament, and pubofemoral ligament. Tension in the anterior portion of the gluteus medius, the gluteus minimus, the adductor magnus and longus, and the pectineus muscles also may contribute to the firm end-feel.

GONIOMETER ALIGNMENT (Figs. 4-17 and 4-18)

The alignment is the same as for measuring medial rotation of the hip.

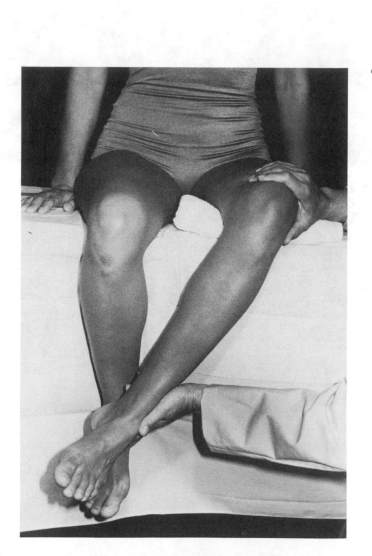

FIGURE 4-16. The subject's left lower extremity is shown at the end of the ROM of hip lateral rotation. The examiner places her right hand on the subject's distal femur to prevent both hip flexion and hip abduction. The subject assists with stabilization by placing her hands on the supporting surface and shifting her weight over her left hip. The subject flexes her right knee to allow the left lower extremity to complete the ROM.

MEASUREMENT OF JOINT MOTION: A GUIDE TO GONIOMETRY

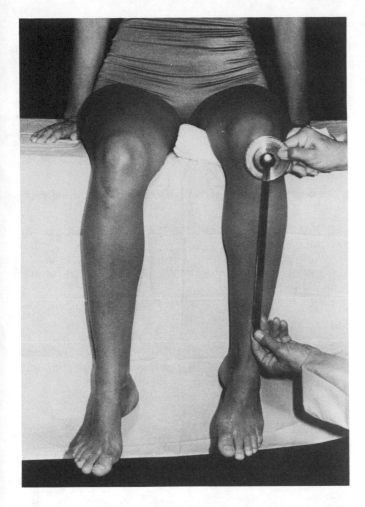

FIGURE 4-17. In the starting position for measuring lateral hip rotation, goniometer alignment is the same as for measuring medial hip rotation.

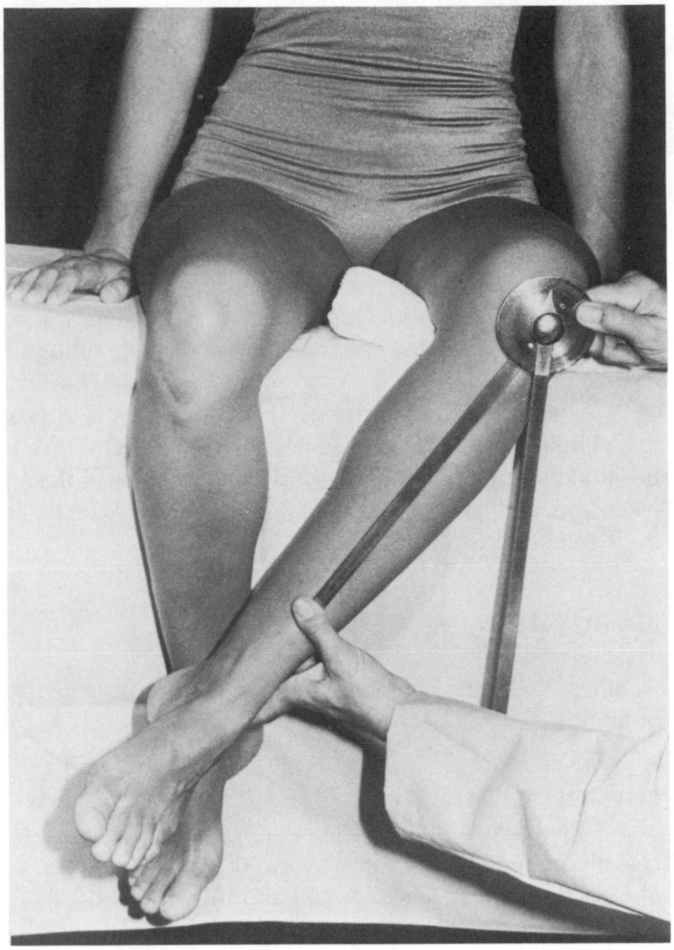

FIGURE 4-18. At the end of the ROM, the examiner uses her left hand to support the subject's leg and to maintain alignment of the distal goniometer arm. When the examiner holds the goniometer body, the freely movable proximal arm hangs so that it is perpendicular to the floor.

THE KNEE: TIBIOFEMORAL JOINT

FLEXION

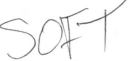

Motion occurs in the sagittal plane around a coronal axis.

RECOMMENDED TESTING POSITION

For the best stabilization, position the subject prone with the hip in 0 degrees of abduction, adduction, flexion, extension, and rotation. The foot is over the edge of the supporting surface.

As an alternative, if the rectus femoris muscle appears to be limiting the range of knee flexion, the subject should be positioned supine. Initially, the hip is in 0 degrees of flexion, extension, abduction, and adduction, but as the knee begins to flex, the hip is also flexed.

STABILIZATION (Fig. 4-19)

Stabilize the femur to prevent rotation, flexion, or extension of the hip.

PHYSIOLOGIC END-FEEL

Usually the end-feel is soft because of contact between the muscle bulk of the posterior calf and thigh, or between the heel and the buttocks. Sometimes the end-feel is firm because of tension in the rectus femoris muscle.

GONIOMETER ALIGNMENT (Figs. 4-20 and 4-21)

1. Center the fulcrum of the goniometer over the lateral epicondyle of the femur.
2. Align the proximal arm with the lateral midline of the femur, using the greater trochanter for reference.
3. Align the distal arm with the lateral midline of the fibula, using the lateral malleolus for reference.

EXTENSION

Motion occurs in the sagittal plane around a coronal axis.

RECOMMENDED TESTING AND GONIOMETER ALIGNMENT

The testing position and alignment are the same as for measuring knee flexion.

STABILIZATION

Stabilize the femur to prevent rotation, flexion, or extension of the hip. If the hip is flexed, tension in the hamstring muscles may restrict the motion.

PHYSIOLOGIC END-FEEL

The end-feel is firm because of tension in the posterior joint capsule, the oblique and arcuate popliteal ligaments, collateral ligaments, and the anterior and posterior cruciate ligaments.

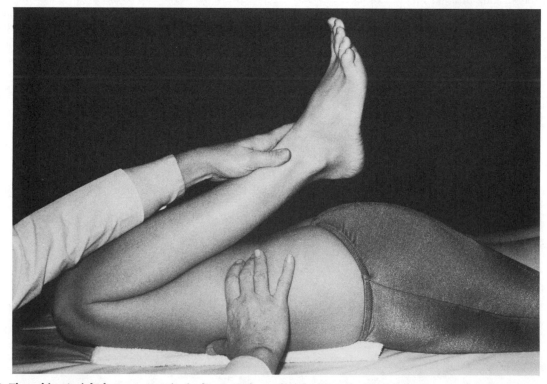

FIGURE 4-19. The subject's right lower extremity is shown at the end of the knee flexion ROM. The examiner's right hand is positioned on the proximal rather than the distal femur so that the posterior surfaces of the distal thigh and lower leg may make contact without interference. The amount of soft tissue that is present on the posterior surfaces of the lower extremity and its degree of compressibility partly determine the extent of the ROM.

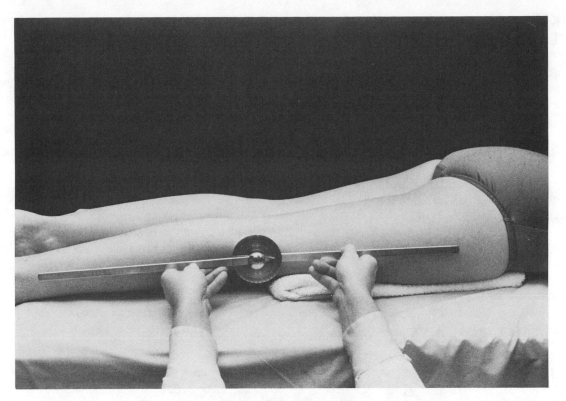

FIGURE 4-20. In the starting position for measuring knee flexion, the subject is in the prone position. A towel is placed under the subject's thigh and the foot is off the supporting surface to allow the knee to fully extend. The examiner either kneels or sits on a stool in order to align and read the goniometer at eye level.

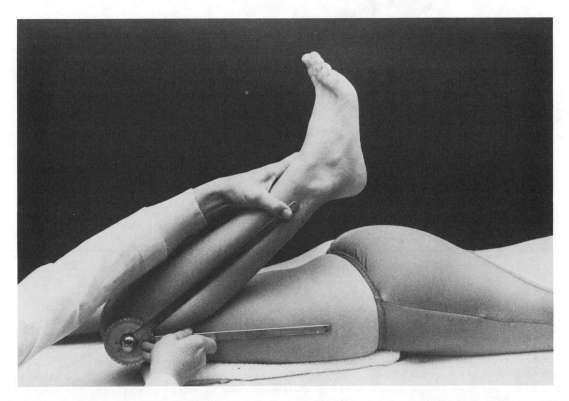

FIGURE 4-21. At the end of the knee flexion ROM, the examiner's right hand aligns the proximal goniometeter arm with the lateral midline of the subject's thigh, using the greater trochanter as a reference point. The subject's upper thigh is exposed so that the greater trochanter may be palpated. The examiner uses her left hand to maintain knee flexion and to keep the distal goniometer arm aligned along the lateral midline of the lower leg.

THE ANKLE: TALOCRURAL JOINT

DORSIFLEXION

Motion occurs in the sagittal plane around a coronal axis.

RECOMMENDED TESTING POSITION

Position the subject sitting or supine, with knee flexed at least 30 degrees. The foot is positioned in 0 degrees of inversion and eversion.

STABILIZATION (Fig. 4-22)

Stabilize the tibia and fibula to prevent knee motion and hip rotation.

PHYSIOLOGIC END-FEEL

The end-feel is firm because of tension in the posterior joint capsule, Achilles tendon, the posterior portion of the deltoid ligament, posterior talofibular ligament, and calcaneofibular ligament.

GONIOMETER ALIGNMENT (Figs. 4-23 and 4-24)

1. Center the fulcrum of the goniometer over the lateral aspect of the lateral malleolus.
2. Align the proximal arm with the lateral midline of the fibula, using the head of the fibula for reference.
3. Align the distal arm parallel to the lateral aspect of the fifth metatarsal. Although it is usually easier to palpate and align the distal arm parallel to the fifth metatarsal, as an alternative, the distal arm can be aligned parallel to the inferior aspect of the calcaneus.

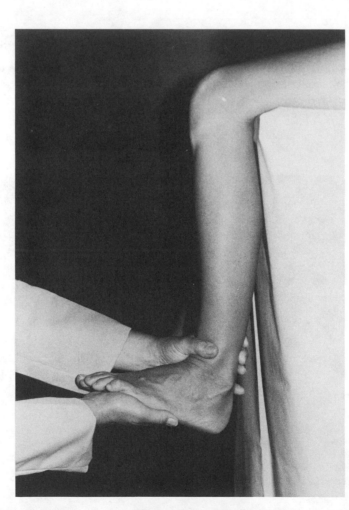

FIGURE 4-22. The subject's left ankle is shown at the end of the dorsiflexion ROM. The examiner holds the distal portion of the lower leg with her left hand to prevent knee motion. The examiner's right hand pushes upward on the plantar surface of the subject's foot to produce dorsiflexion. The examiner avoids pushing on the toes. A considerable amount of upward force is necessary because of the resistance offered by the gastrocnemius and soleus muscles. The amount of force that is necessary to overcome tension in the Achilles tendon varies from subject to subject. Often a comparison between the active and passive ranges of motion helps one to determine the amount of upward force that must be exerted to complete the passive ROM in dorsiflexion for a particular individual.

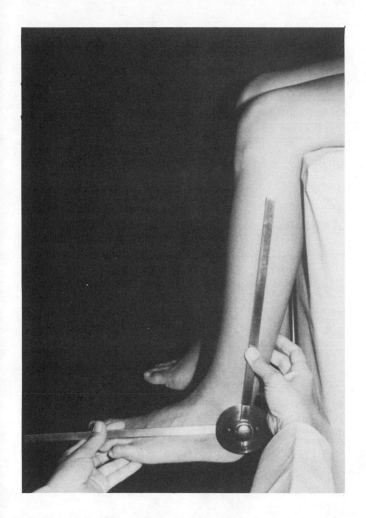

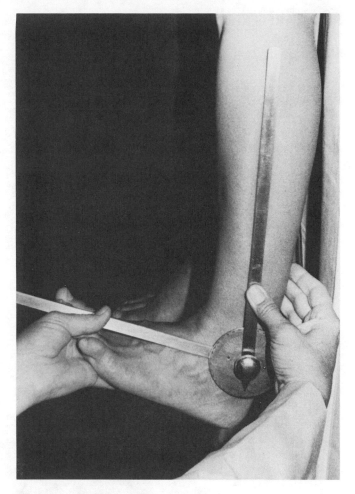

FIGURE 4-23. In the starting position for measuring dorsiflexion, the proximal arm of the goniometer is aligned with the lateral midline of the lower leg using the head of the fibula as a reference point. The examiner aligns the distal goniometer arm parallel to the fifth metatarsal. The ankle is positioned so that the goniometer is at 90 degrees. Therefore, the same adjustments in recording are made as for hip abduction and hip adduction. The examiner sits on a stool or kneels so that the goniometer may be both aligned and read at eye level.

FIGURE 4-24. At the end of dorsiflexion, the examiner's right hand aligns the proximal goniometer arm, while the examiner's left hand maintains dorsiflexion and alignment of the distal goniometer arm.

PLANTARFLEXION

Motion occurs in the sagittal plane around a coronal axis.

RECOMMENDED TESTING POSITION

The testing position and alignment are the same as for ankle dorsiflexion.

STABILIZATION (Fig. 4-25)

Stabilize the tibia and fibula to prevent knee flexion and hip rotation.

PHYSIOLOGIC END-FEEL

Usually the end-feel is firm because of tension in the anterior joint capsule, the anterior portion of the deltoid ligament, the anterior talofibular ligament, and the tibialis anterior, extensor hallucis longus, and extensor digitorum longus muscles. The end-feel may be hard because of contact between the posterior tubercles of the talus and the posterior margin of the tibia.

GONIOMETER ALIGNMENT (Figs. 4-26 and 4-27)

The alignment is the same as for ankle dorsiflexion.

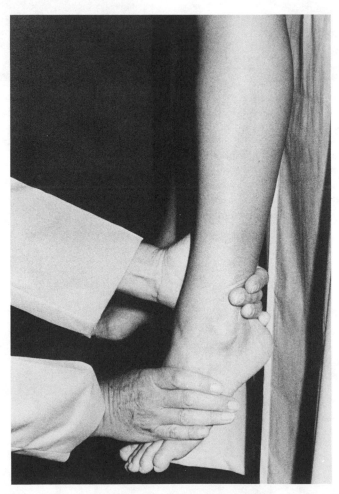

FIGURE 4-25. The subject's left ankle is shown at the end of the plantarflexion ROM. The examiner holds the subject's lower leg to prevent knee flexion. The examiner's right hand pushes downward on the dorsum of the subject's foot to produce plantarflexion. No force is exerted on the subject's toes, and the examiner is careful to avoid pushing the ankle into inversion or eversion.

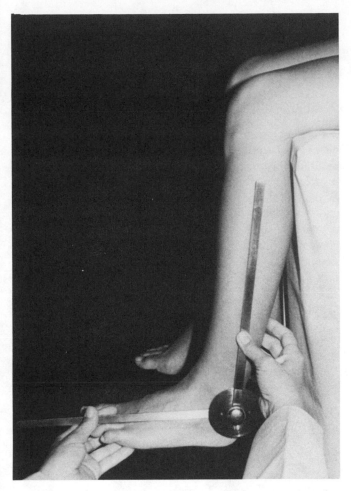

FIGURE 4-26. Initial goniometer alignment for measuring plantarflexion is the same as for measuring dorsiflexion.

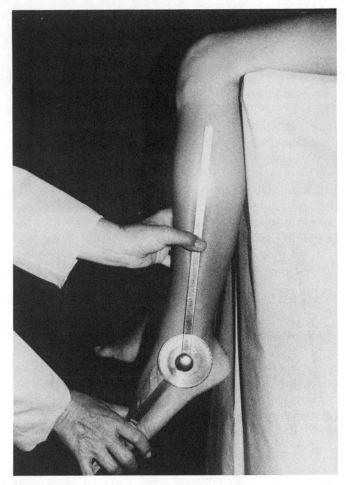

FIGURE 4-27. At the end of plantarflexion, the examiner uses her right hand to maintain plantarflexion and to align the distal goniometer arm. The examiner grasps the dorsum and sides of the foot to avoid exerting pressure on the toes.

THE FOOT: TARSAL JOINTS

INVERSION

This motion is a combination of supination, adduction, and plantarflexion occurring in varying degrees at the subtalar, transverse tarsal (talocalcaneonavicular and calcaneocuboid), cuboideonavicular, cuneonavicular, intercuneiform, cuneocuboid, tarsometatarsal, and intermetatarsal joints. The functional ability of the foot to adapt to the ground and to absorb contact forces depends upon the combined movement in all of these joints. A method of measuring the combined movements at these joints is presented below. Because of the uniaxial limitations of the goniometer, inversion is measured in the frontal plane around an anterior-posterior axis. Methods for measuring inversion of the hindfoot and mid- and forefoot are included in the sections on the subtalar and transverse tarsal joints.

RECOMMENDED TESTING POSITION

Position the subject sitting with the knee flexed to 90 degrees and the lower leg over the edge of the supporting surface. The hip is in 0 degrees of rotation, adduction, and abduction. Alternatively, it is possible to position the subject supine with the foot over the supporting surface.

STABILIZATION (Fig. 4-28)

Stabilize the tibia and fibula to prevent medial rotation and extension of the knee and lateral rotation and abduction of the hip.

PHYSIOLOGIC END-FEEL

The end-feel is firm because of tension in the joint capsules, the anterior and posterior talofibular ligament, the calcaneofibular ligament, anterior, posterior, lateral, and interosseous talocalcaneal ligaments, the dorsal calcaneal ligaments, the dorsal calcaneocuboid ligament, dorsal talonavicular ligament, the lateral band of the bifurcate ligament, transverse metatarsal ligament, various dorsal, plantar, and interosseous ligaments of the cuboideonavicular, cuneonavicular, intercuneiform, cuneocuboid, tarsometatarsal, and intermetatarsal joints, and the peroneus longus and brevis muscles.

GONIOMETER ALIGNMENT (Figs. 4-29 and 4-30)

1. Center the fulcrum of the goniometer over the anterior aspect of the ankle midway between the malleoli.
2. Align the proximal arm of the goniometer with the anterior midline of the lower leg, using the crest of the tibia for reference.
3. Align the distal arm with the anterior midline of the second metatarsal.

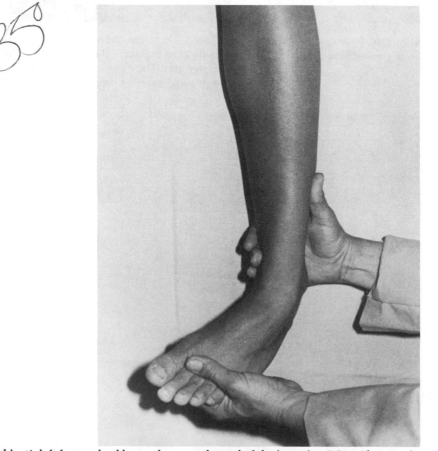

FIGURE 4-28. The subject's left foot and ankle are shown at the end of the inversion ROM. The examiner's right hand grasps the subject's distal lower leg to prevent both knee and hip motion. The examiner's left hand maintains inversion. Because inversion includes supination, adduction, and plantarflexion, the subject's ankle moves in these three directions.

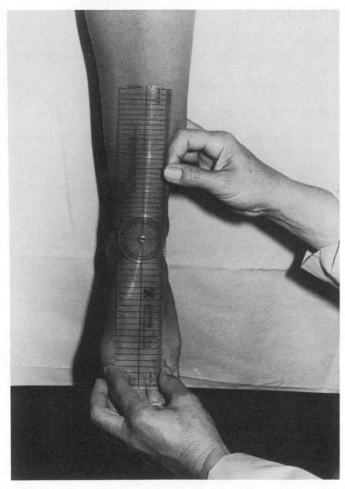 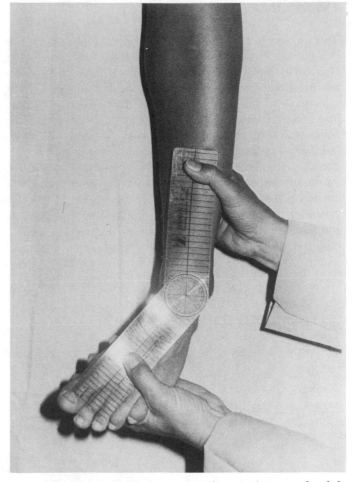

FIGURE 4-29. In the starting position for measuring inversion, the body of the plastic full-circle goniometer is positioned midway between the two malleoli. The flexibility of the plastic goniometer makes this particular instrument easier to use for measuring inversion than a metal goniometer. The examiner aligns the proximal goniometer arm along the crest of the tibia and the distal arm with the second metatarsal.

FIGURE 4-30. At the end of inversion, the examiner uses her left hand to maintain inversion and to align the distal goniometer arm.

EVERSION

This motion is a combination of pronation, abduction, and dorsiflexion occurring in varying degrees at the subtalar, transverse tarsal (talocalcaneonavicular and calcaneocuboid), cuboideonavicular, cuneonavicular, intercuneiform, cuneocuboid, and tarsometatarsal and intermetatarsal joints. The functional ability of the foot to adapt to the ground and to absorb contact forces depends upon the combined movement of all of these joints. A method for measuring the combined movements at these joints is presented below. Because of the uniaxial limitations of the goniometer, this motion is measured in the frontal plane around an anterior-posterior axis. Methods for measuring eversion isolated to the hindfoot and mid- and forefoot are included in the sections on the subtalar and transverse tarsal joints.

RECOMMENDED TESTING POSITION

The testing position is the same as for measuring inversion of the foot.

STABILIZATION (Fig. 4-31)

Stabilize the tibia and fibula to prevent lateral rotation and flexion of the knee and medial rotation and adduction of the hip.

PHYSIOLOGIC END-FEEL 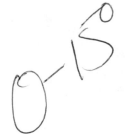 *Hard/Firm*

The end-feel may be hard because of contact between the calcaneus and the floor of the sinus tarsi. In some cases, the end-feel may be firm because of tension in the joint capsules, the deltoid ligament, the medial talocalcaneal ligament, the plantar calcaneonavicular and calcaneocuboid ligaments, the dorsal talonavicular ligament, the medial band of the bifurcated ligament, the transverse metatarsal ligament, various dorsal, plantar, and interosseous ligaments of the cuboideonavicular, cuneonavicular, intercuneiform, cuneocuboid, tarsometatarsal, and intermetatarsal joints, and the tibialis posterior muscle.

GONIOMETER ALIGNMENT (Figs. 4-32 and 4-33)

The alignment is the same as for measuring inversion of the foot.

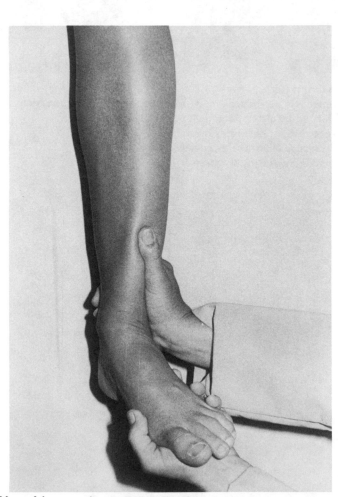

FIGURE 4-31. The subject's left ankle and foot are shown at the end of the ROM in eversion. The examiner uses her right hand on the subject's distal lower leg to prevent both knee flexion and lateral rotation. The examiner's left hand is maintaining eversion.

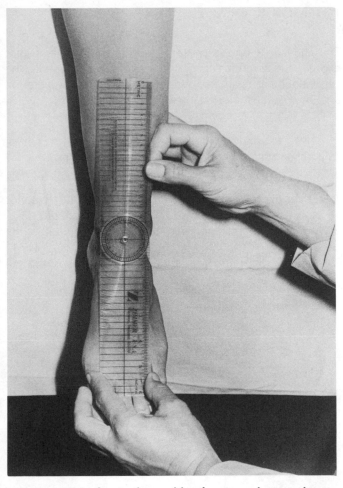 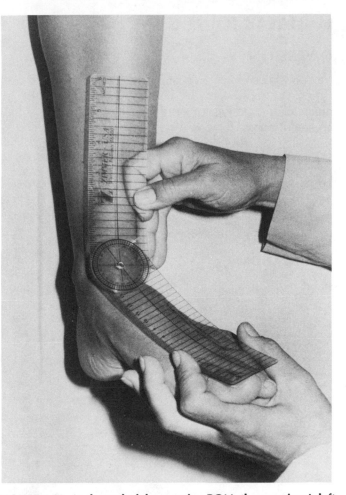

FIGURE 4-32. In the starting position for measuring eversion, goniometer alignment is the same as for measuring inversion.

FIGURE 4-33. At the end of the eversion ROM, the examiner's left hand maintains eversion and keeps the distal goniometer arm aligned with the subject's second metatarsal. The examiner's right hand maintains the alignment of the proximal goniometer arm with the crest of the tibia. Because eversion includes pronation, abduction, and dorsiflexion the subject's foot is moved in these three directions.

SUBTALAR JOINT (HINDFOOT)

INVERSION

Motion is a combination of supination, adduction, and plantarflexion. Because of the uniaxial limitations of the goniometer, this motion is measured in the frontal plane around an anterior-posterior axis.

RECOMMENDED TESTING POSITION

Position the subject prone with the hip in 0 degrees of flexion, extension, abduction, adduction, and rotation. The knee is in 0 degrees of flexion and extension. The foot is placed over the edge of the supporting surface.

STABILIZATION (Fig. 4-34)

Stabilize the tibia and fibula to prevent hip and knee motion.

PHYSIOLOGIC END-FEEL

The end-feel is firm because of tension in the lateral joint capsule, the anterior and posterior talofibular ligaments, the calcaneofibular ligament, and the lateral, posterior, anterior, and interosseous talocalcaneal ligaments.

GONIOMETER ALIGNMENT (Figs. 4-35 and 4-36)

1. Center the fulcrum of the goniometer over the posterior aspect of the ankle midway between the malleoli.
2. Align the proximal arm with the posterior midline of the lower leg.
3. Align the distal arm with the posterior midline of the calcaneus.

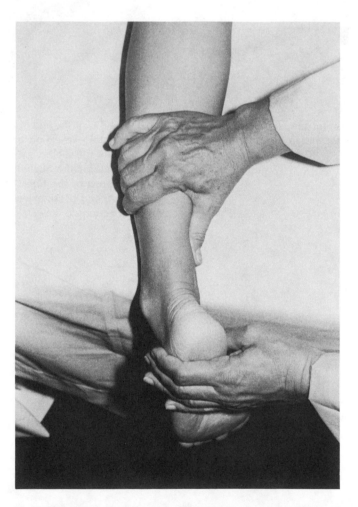

FIGURE 4-34. The subject's left lower extremity is shown at the end of the subtalar inversion ROM. The subject is in a prone position with her left foot and ankle extended over the edge of the supporting surface. The examiner is stabilizing the subject's lower leg to prevent medial knee rotation and hip adduction. The examiner's left hand pulls the subject's calcaneus medially to produce subtalar inversion. The examiner avoids pushing on the forefoot.

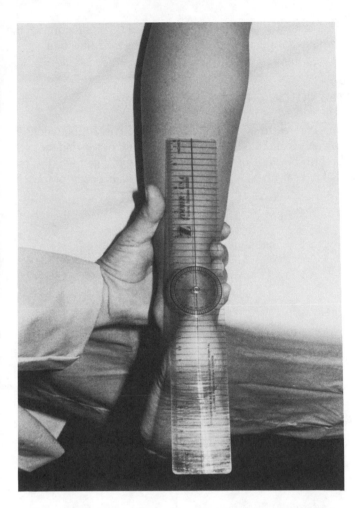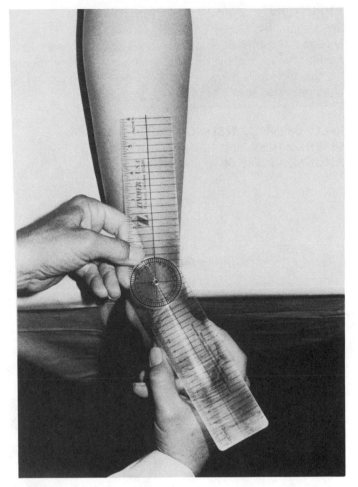

FIGURE 4-35. In the starting position for measuring subtalar inversion, the goniometer body is centered midway between the two malleoli. The proximal goniometer arm is aligned along the midline of the posterior lower leg. The distal arm is aligned with the posterior midline of the calcaneus. Normally, the examiner's right hand would be holding the distal goniometer arm, but this is not being done here, for purposes of this photograph.

FIGURE 4-36. At the end of subtalar inversion, the examiner's right hand maintains inversion and keeps the distal goniometer arm in alignment. The examiner uses her left hand to maintain alignment of the proximal arm.

EVERSION

Motion is a combination of pronation, abduction, and dorsiflexion. Because of the uniaxial limitations of the goniometer, this motion is measured in the frontal plane around an anterior-posterior axis.

RECOMMENDED TESTING POSITION AND STABILIZATION (Fig. 4-37) AND GONIOMETER ALIGNMENT (Figs. 4-38 and 4-39)

The testing position, stabilization, and alignment are the same as for measuring inversion at the subtalar joint.

PHYSIOLOGIC END-FEEL

The end-feel may be hard because of contact between the calcaneus and the floor of the sinus tarsi; or the end-feel may be firm because of tension in the deltoid ligament, the medial talocalcaneal ligament, and the tibialis posterior muscle.

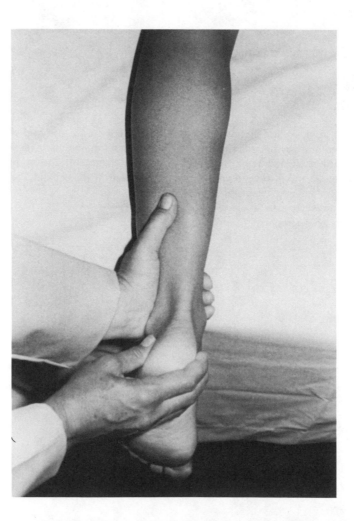

FIGURE 4-37. The subject's left lower extremity is shown at the end of subtalar eversion. One can observe that this subject's eversion ROM is more limited than her subtalar inversion ROM. The examiner stabilizes the subject's distal tibia and fibula to prevent knee lateral rotation and hip abduction. The examiner's right hand maintains subtalar eversion by pulling the calcaneus laterally.

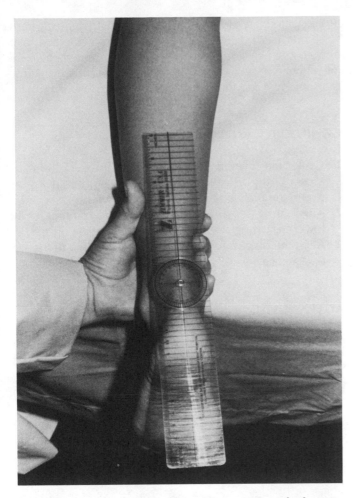

FIGURE 4-38. In the starting position for measuring subtalar eversion, the goniometer alignment is the same as for measuring subtalar inversion.

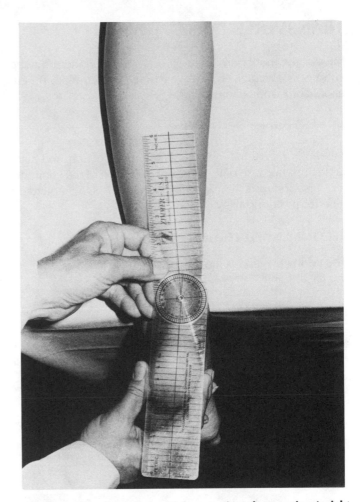

FIGURE 4-39. At the end of subtalar eversion, the examiner's right hand maintains eversion and keeps the distal goniometer arm aligned with the midline of the calcaneus. The examiner's left hand maintains alignment of the proximal arm with the midline of the lower leg.

TRANSVERSE TARSAL JOINT

Most of the motion in the midfoot and forefoot occurs at the cuboideonavicular, cuneonavicular, intercuneiform, cuneocuboid, and tarsometatarsal joints.

INVERSION

Motion is a combination of supination, adduction, and plantarflexion. Because of the uniaxial limitation of the goniometer, this motion is measured in the frontal plane around an anterior-posterior axis.

RECOMMENDED TESTING POSITION

The testing position is the same as for measuring inversion at the tarsal joints.

STABILIZATION (Fig. 4-40)

Stabilize the calcaneus and talus to prevent dorsiflexion of the ankle and inversion of the subtalar joint.

PHYSIOLOGIC END-FEEL

The end-feel is firm because of tension in the joint capsules, the dorsal calcaneocuboid ligament, the dorsal talonavicular ligament, the lateral band of the bifurcated ligament, transverse metatarsal ligament, various dorsal, plantar, and interosseous ligaments of the cuboideonavicular, cuneonavicular, intercuneiform, cuneocuboid, tarsometatarsal, and intermetatarsal joints; and the peroneus longus and brevis muscles.

GONIOMETER ALIGNMENT (Figs. 4-41 and 4-42)

1. Center the fulcrum of the goniometer over the anterior aspect of the ankle slightly distal to a point midway between the malleoli.
2. Align the proximal arm with the anterior midline of the lower leg, using the crest of the tibia for reference.
3. Align the distal arm with the anterior midline of the second metatarsal.

ALTERNATIVE GONIOMETER ALIGNMENT
(Figs. 4-43 and 4-44)

1. Place the fulcrum of the goniometer at the lateral aspect of the fifth metatarsal head.
2. Align the proximal arm parallel to the anterior midline of the lower leg.
3. Align the distal arm with the plantar aspect of the first through fifth metatarsal heads.

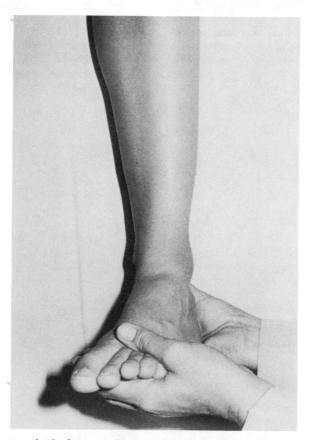

FIGURE 4-40. The subject's left lower extremity is shown at the end of transverse tarsal inversion ROM. The examiner's right hand cups the calcaneus to prevent subtalar inversion. The examiner's left hand pushes the forefoot medially to produce inversion. The examiner's left hand grasps the subject's metatarsals rather than the subject's toes. Notice that the extent of the ROM is very small.

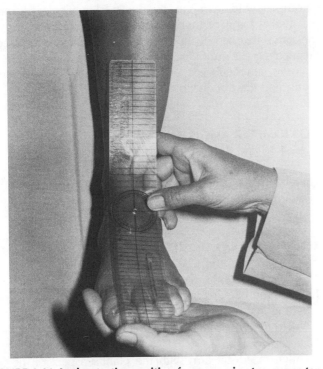

FIGURE 4-41. In the starting position for measuring transverse tarsal inversion, the goniometer alignment is similar to the alignment used for measuring inversion (see Fig. 4-29). In Figure 4-29, the body of the goniometer is placed between the two malleoli, whereas when measuring transverse tarsal inversion, the goniometer body is placed distal to the malleoli on the dorsum of the foot.

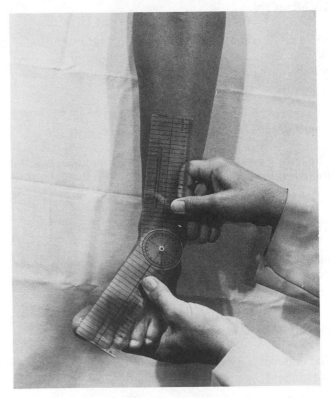

FIGURE 4-42. At the end of transverse tarsal inversion, the examiner's left hand maintains inversion and holds the distal goniometer aligned along the second metatarsal. The examiner's right hand maintains alignment of the proximal goniometer arm.

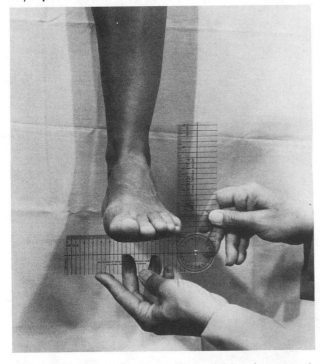

FIGURE 4-43. In the alternative starting position for measuring transverse tarsal inversion, the examiner aligns the proximal goniometer arm so that it is perpendicular to the subject's tibia. The examiner positions the distal goniometer arm across the plantar surface of the subject's foot on level with the heads of the metatarsals. This goniometer alignment places the goniometer at 90 degrees, which is the 0 starting position. Therefore, the recording must be adjusted in the same way it was adjusted in hip abduction and adduction.

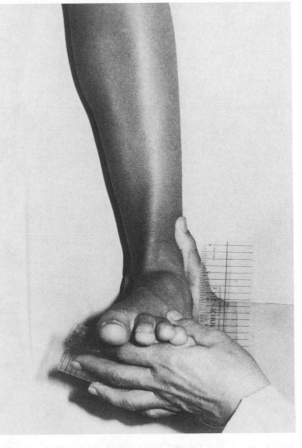

FIGURE 4-44. At the end of the transverse tarsal inversion ROM, the examiner uses her left hand to maintain inversion and to keep the distal goniometer arm aligned.

EVERSION

Motion is a combination of pronation, abduction, and dorsiflexion. Because of the uniaxial limitations of the goniometer, this motion is measured in the frontal plane around an anterior-posterior axis.

RECOMMENDED TESTING POSITION

The testing position is the same as for measuring eversion at the tarsal joints.

STABILIZATION (Fig. 4-45)

Stabilize the calcaneus and talus to prevent plantarflexion of the ankle and eversion of the subtalar joint.

PHYSIOLOGIC END-FEEL

The end-feel is firm because of tension in the joint capsules, the deltoid ligament, the plantar calcaneonavicular and calcaneocuboid ligaments, the dorsal talonavicular ligament, the medial band of the bifurcated ligament, the transverse metatarsal ligament, various dorsal, plantar, and interosseous ligaments of the cuboideonavicular, cuneonavicular, intercuneiform, cuneocuboid, tarsometatarsal, and intermetatarsal joints, and the tibialis posterior muscle.

GONIOMETER ALIGNMENT
(Figs. 4-46 and 4-47)

The alignment is the same as for measuring inversion at the transverse tarsal joint.

ALTERNATIVE GONIOMETER ALIGNMENT
(Figs. 4-48 and 4-49)

1. Place the fulcrum of the goniometer at the medial aspect of the first metatarsal head.
2. Align the proximal arm parallel to the anterior midline of the lower leg.
3. Align the distal arm with the plantar aspect of the first through fifth metatarsal heads.

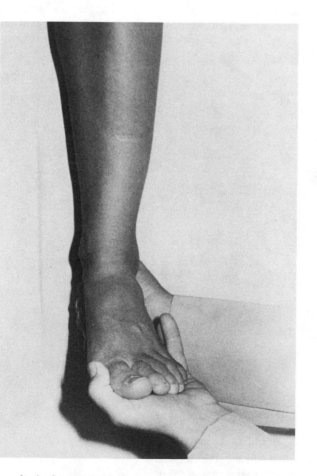

FIGURE 4-45. The subject's left lower extremity is shown at the end of the transverse tarsal eversion ROM. The examiner's right hand is stabilizing the calcaneus to prevent subtalar eversion. As can be seen in the photograph, only a small amount of motion is available.

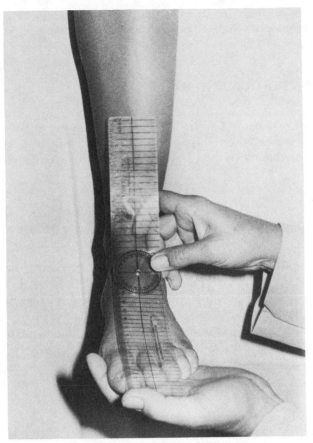

FIGURE 4-46. In the starting position for measuring transverse tarsal eversion, goniometer alignment is the same as that used for measuring transverse tarsal inversion.

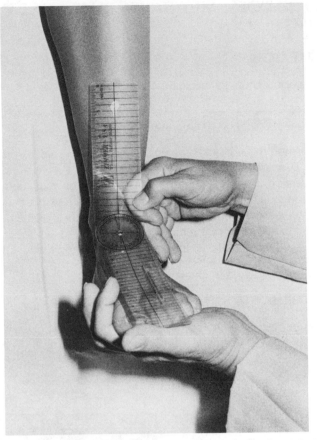

FIGURE 4-47. At the end of the transverse tarsal eversion ROM, the examiner's left hand maintains eversion and holds the distal goniometer arm aligned with the second metatarsal.

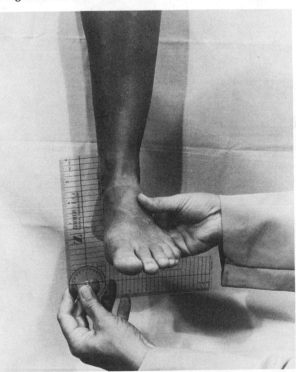

FIGURE 4-48. Goniometer alignment in the alternative starting position for measuring transverse tarsal eversion is similar to that used for measuring transverse tarsal inversion (see Fig. 4-43). However, when measuring eversion, the goniometer is positioned on the medial rather than on the lateral aspect of the foot.

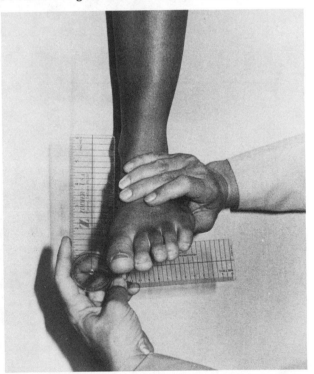

FIGURE 4-49. At the end of the ROM, the examiner's right hand maintains eversion, while her left hand aligns the goniometer. Because the subject is sitting on a table, the examiner sits on a low stool so that she is able to align and read the goniometer at eye level.

THE TOES: METATARSOPHALANGEAL (MTP) JOINT

FLEXION

Motion occurs in the sagittal plane around a coronal axis.

RECOMMENDED TESTING POSITION

Position the subject supine or sitting, with the ankle and foot in 0 degrees of dorsiflexion, plantarflexion, inversion, and eversion. The MTP joint is in 0 degrees of abduction and adduction. The interphalangeal (IP) joints are positioned in 0 degrees of flexion and extension. (If the ankle is plantarflexed and the IP joints of the toe being tested are flexed, tension in the extensor hallucis longus or extensor digitorum longus muscle will restrict the motion.)

STABILIZATION (Fig. 4-50)

Stabilize the metatarsal to prevent plantarflexion of the ankle and inversion or eversion of the foot. Do not hold the MTP joints of the other toes in extension, as tension in the transverse metatarsal ligament will restrict the motion.

PHYSIOLOGIC END-FEEL

The end-feel is firm because of tension in the dorsal joint capsule and the collateral ligaments. Tension in the extensor digitorum brevis muscle may contribute to the firm end-feel.

GONIOMETER ALIGNMENT (Figs. 4-51 and 4-52)

1. Center the fulcrum of the goniometer over the dorsal aspect of the MTP joint.
2. Align the proximal arm over the dorsal midline of the metatarsal.
3. Align the distal arm over the dorsal midline of the proximal phalanx.

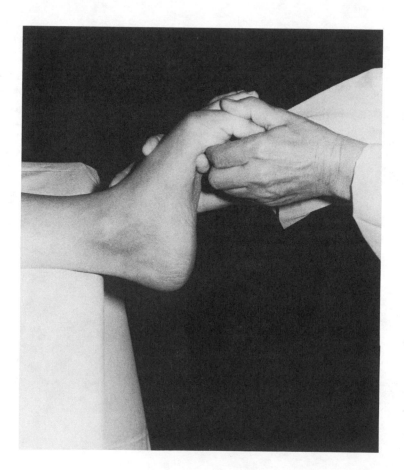

FIGURE 4-50. The subject's left first metatarsophalangeal joint is shown at the end of the flexion ROM. The subject is lying in a supine position with her foot and ankle extending over the edge of the supporting surface. However, the subject's foot may be allowed to rest on the supporting surface. The examiner's right thumb is placed across the metatarsals to prevent plantarflexion. The examiner's left hand maintains the first metatarsophalangeal joint in flexion.

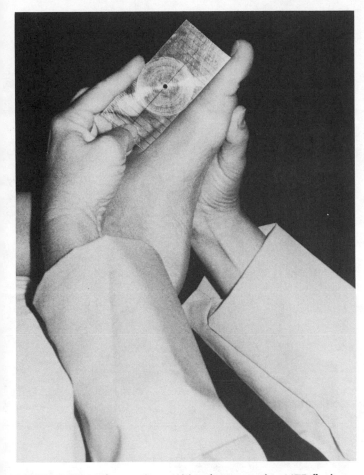 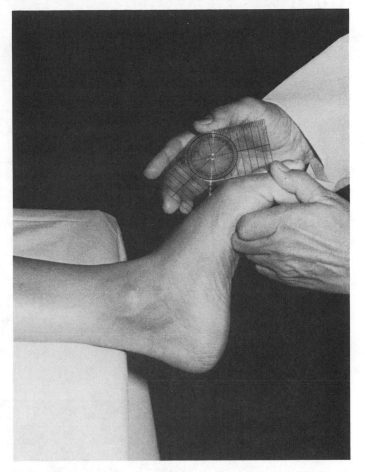

FIGURE 4-51. In the starting position for measuring MTP flexion, the arms of the goniometer are placed on the dorsal surface of the metatarsal and proximal phalanx. A portion of the arms of the goniometer has been cut off to accommodate the relatively small proximal and distal joint segments.

FIGURE 4-52. At the end of the ROM the examiner's right hand aligns the goniometer, while the examiner's left hand maintains MTP flexion.

EXTENSION

Motion occurs in the sagittal plane around a coronal axis.

RECOMMENDED TESTING POSITION

The testing position is the same as for measuring flexion of the MTP joint. (If the ankle is dorsiflexed and the IP joints of the toe being tested are extended, tension in the flexor hallucis longus or flexor digitorum longus muscles will restrict the motion. If the IP joints of the toe being tested are in extreme flexion, tension in the lumbricals and interossei muscles may restrict the motion.)

STABILIZATION (Fig. 4-53)

Stabilize the metatarsal to prevent dorsiflexion of the ankle and inversion or eversion of the foot. Do not hold the MTP joints of the other toes in extreme flexion, as tension in the transverse metatarsal ligament will restrict the motion.

PHYSIOLOGIC END-FEEL

The end-feel is firm because of tension in the plantar joint capsule, the plantar pad (plantar fibrocartilaginous plate), and the flexor hallucis brevis, flexor digitorium brevis, and the flexor digiti minimi muscles.

GONIOMETER ALIGNMENT (Figs. 4-54 and 4-55)

The alignment is the same as for measuring flexion of the MTP joint.

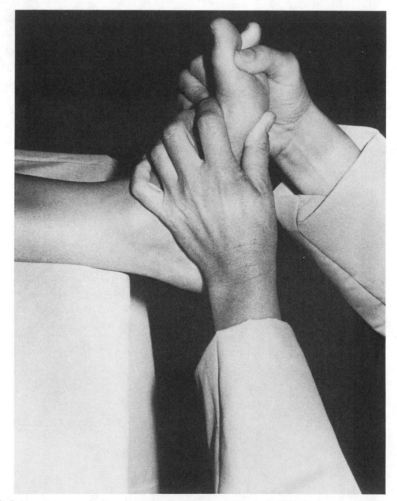

FIGURE 4-53. The subject's left first metatarsophalangeal joint is shown at the end of the extension ROM. The subject's position is the same as for measuring MTP flexion. The examiner's left digits are placed on the dorsum of the foot to prevent dorsiflexion. The examiner uses her right thumb to push the proximal phalanx into extension.

MEASUREMENT OF JOINT MOTION: A GUIDE TO GONIOMETRY

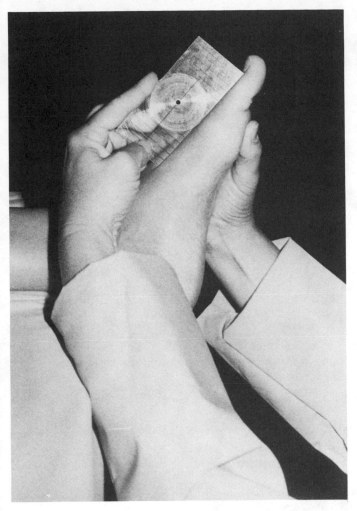

FIGURE 4-54. Goniometer alignment in the starting position for MTP extension is the same as that for measuring MTP flexion.

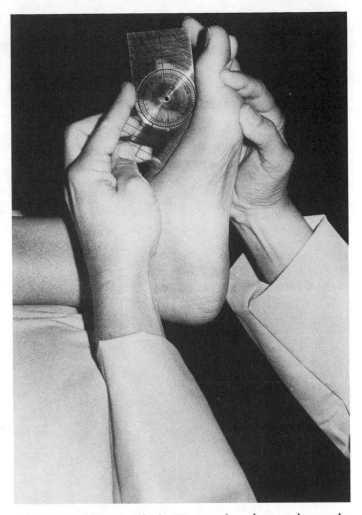

FIGURE 4-55. At the end of MTP extension, the examiner maintains goniometer alignment with her left hand, while she uses her right index finger to maintain extension.

ABDUCTION

Motion occurs in the transverse plane around a vertical axis, when the subject is in anatomic position.

RECOMMENDED TESTING POSITION

Position the subject supine or sitting with the foot in 0 degrees of inversion and eversion. The MTP and IP joints are positioned in 0 degrees of flexion and extension.

STABILIZATION (Fig. 4-56)

Stabilize the metatarsal to prevent inversion or eversion of the foot.

PHYSIOLOGIC END-FEEL

The end-feel is firm because of tension in the joint capsule, the collateral ligaments, the fascia of the web space between the toes, and the adductor hallucis and plantar interossei muscles.

GONIOMETER ALIGNMENT (Figs. 4-57 and 4-58)

1. Center the fulcrum of the goniometer over the dorsal aspect of the MTP joint.
2. Align the proximal arm with the dorsal midline of the metatarsal.
3. Align the distal arm with the dorsal midline of the proximal phalanx.

ADDUCTION

Motion occurs in the transverse plane around a vertical axis, when the subject is in anatomic position.

RECOMMENDED TESTING POSITION, STABILIZATION, AND GONIOMETER ALIGNMENT

The testing position, stabilization, and alignment are the same as for measuring abduction of the MTP joints.

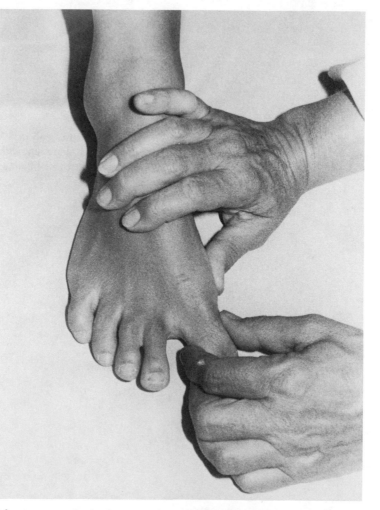

FIGURE 4-56. The subject's right lower extremity is shown at the end of MTP abduction. The examiner's right thumb is being used to prevent transverse tarsal inversion. The examiner's left index finger and thumb are being used to pull the proximal phalanx of the toe into abduction.

MEASUREMENT OF JOINT MOTION: A GUIDE TO GONIOMETRY

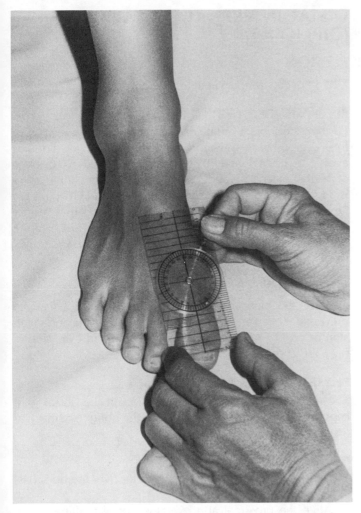

FIGURE 4-57. In the starting position for measuring MTP abduction, the adapted full-circle plastic goniometer is positioned so that the fulcrum is over the MTP joint. The proximal arm is aligned with the first metatarsal. The distal arm is aligned along the midline of the proximal phalanx.

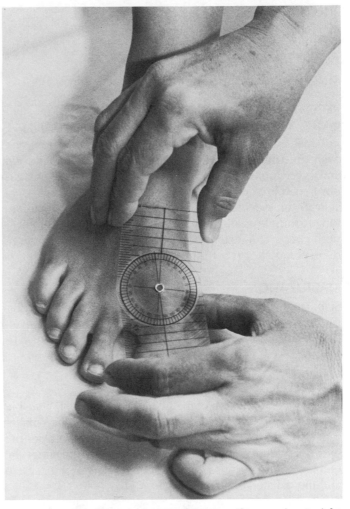

FIGURE 4-58. At the end of MTP abduction, the examiner's right hand maintains alignment of the proximal goniometer arm. The examiner's left hand maintains alignment of the distal goniometer arm and maintains the MTP in abduction.

PROXIMAL INTERPHALANGEAL (PIP) JOINT

FLEXION

Motion occurs in the sagittal plane around a coronal axis.

RECOMMENDED TESTING POSITION

Position the subject supine or sitting, with the ankle and foot in 0 degrees of dorsiflexion, plantarflexion, inversion, and eversion. The MTP joint is positioned in 0 degrees of flexion and extension and abduction and adduction. (If the ankle is positioned in plantarflexion and the MTP joint is flexed, tension in the extensor hallucis longus or extensor digitorum longus muscles will restrict the motion. If the MTP joint is positioned in full extension, tension in the lumbrical and interossei muscles may restrict the motion.)

STABILIZATION

Stabilize the metatarsal and proximal phalanx to prevent dorsiflexion or plantarflexion of the ankle and inversion or eversion of the foot. Avoid flexion and extension of the MTP joint.

PHYSIOLOGIC END-FEEL

The end-feel for flexion of the interphalangeal joint of the big toe and the proximal interphalangeal joints of the smaller toes may be soft because of compression of soft tissues between the plantar surfaces of the phalanges. Sometimes the end-feel is firm because of tension in the dorsal joint capsule and the collateral ligaments.

GONIOMETER ALIGNMENT

1. Center the fulcrum of the goniometer over the dorsal aspect of the interphalangeal joint being tested.
2. Align the proximal arm over the dorsal midline of the proximal phalanx.
3. Align the distal arm over the dorsal midline of the phalanx distal to the joint being tested.

EXTENSION

Motion occurs in the sagittal plane around a coronal axis.

RECOMMENDED TESTING POSITION, STABILIZATION, AND GONIOMETER ALIGNMENT

The testing position, stabilization, and alignment are the same as for measuring flexion of the proximal interphalangeal joints. (If the ankle is positioned in dorsiflexion and the MTP joint is extended, tension in the flexor hallucis longus and brevis muscles and flexor digitorum longus and brevis muscles will restrict the motion.)

PHYSIOLOGIC END-FEEL

The end-feel is firm because of tension in the plantar joint capsule and plantar pad (plantar fibrocartilaginous plate).

DISTAL INTERPHALANGEAL (DIP) JOINT

FLEXION

Motion occurs in the sagittal plane around a coronal axis.

RECOMMENDED TESTING POSITION

Position the subject supine or sitting, with the ankle and foot in 0 degrees of dorsiflexion, plantarflexion, inversion, and eversion. The MTP and PIP joints are positioned in 0 degrees of flexion, extension, abduction, and adduction. (If the ankle is positioned in plantarflexion and the MTP and PIP joints are flexed, tension in the extensor digitorum longus may restrict the motion. If the MTP and PIP joints are held in extreme extension, additional tension in the oblique retinacular ligament will restrict the motion.)

STABILIZATION

Stabilize the metatarsal, proximal, and middle phalanx to prevent dorsiflexion or plantarflexion of the ankle and inversion or eversion of the foot. Avoid flexion and extension of the MTP and PIP joints of the toe being tested.

PHYSIOLOGIC END-FEEL

The end-feel is firm because of tension in the dorsal joint capsule, the collateral ligaments, and the oblique retinacular ligament.

GONIOMETER ALIGNMENT

1. Center the fulcrum of the goniometer over the dorsal aspect of the DIP joint.
2. Align the proximal arm over the dorsal midline of the middle phalanx.
3. Align the distal arm over the dorsal midline of the distal phalanx.

EXTENSION

Motion occurs in the sagittal plane around a coronal axis.

RECOMMENDED TESTING POSITION

The testing position is the same as for flexion of the DIP joints of the toes. (If the ankle is positioned in dorsiflexion and the MCP and PIP joints are fully extended, tension in the flexor digitorum longus, lumbricals, and interossei muscles will restrict the motion.)

STABILIZATION

Stabilize the metatarsal, proximal, and middle phalanx to prevent dorsiflexion or plantarflexion of the ankle and inversion or eversion of the foot. Avoid extreme extension of the MTP and PIP joints of the toe being tested.

PHYSIOLOGIC END-FEEL

The end-feel is firm because of tension in the plantar joint capsule and the plantar pad (plantar fibrocartilaginous plate).

GONIOMETER ALIGNMENT

The alignment is the same as for DIP flexion of the toes.

TESTING OF THE SPINE
AND TEMPOROMANDIBULAR JOINT

OBJECTIVES

Upon completion of this chapter the reader will be able to:

1. Identify:
   the appropriate planes and axes for each spinal motion

2. Describe:
   the recommended testing positions for motions of the spine

3. Perform a goniometric evaluation of the cervical spine including:
   a clear explanation of the testing procedure
   positioning of the subject in a recommended testing position
   adequate stabilization of the proximal joint component
   a correct determination of the end of the range of motion
   palpation of the correct bony landmarks
   correct alignment of the goniometer
   correct reading and recording

4. Perform an evaluation of the cervical, thoracic, and lumbar spine using a tape measure.

5. Perform an evaluation of the temporomandibular joint, using either a tape measure or a ruler.

This chapter presents common clinical techniques for measuring gross motions of the cervical, thoracic, and lumbar spine. Evaluation of the ROM and end-feels of individual facet joints of the spine are not included.

CERVICAL SPINE

FLEXION

Motion occurs in the sagittal plane around a coronal axis.

RECOMMENDED TESTING POSITION

Position the subject sitting, with the thoracic and lumbar spine well supported by the back of a chair. The cervical spine is positioned in 0 degrees of rotation and lateral flex-

ion. A tongue depressor can be held between the teeth for reference.

STABILIZATION (Fig. 5-1)

The shoulder girdle is stabilized to prevent flexion of the thoracic and lumbar spine. Usually, the stabilization is achieved through the cooperation of the patient and support from the back of the chair.

GONIOMETER ALIGNMENT (Figs. 5-2 and 5-3)

1. Center the fulcrum of the goniometer over the external auditory meatus.

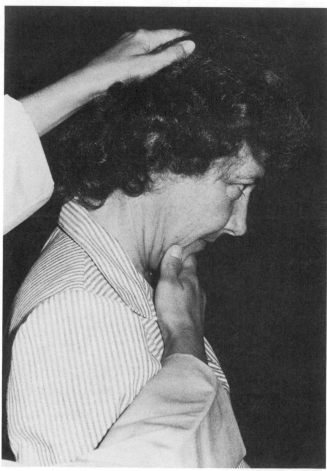

FIGURE 5-1. The subject is shown at the end of the cervical flexion ROM. The examiner's left hand pushes gently on the posterior aspect of the subject's head to maintain cervical flexion. At the same time, the examiner's right hand pulls the subject's chin towards her chest. The examiner's right arm is placed across the subject's chest to prevent thoracic and lumbar spine flexion.

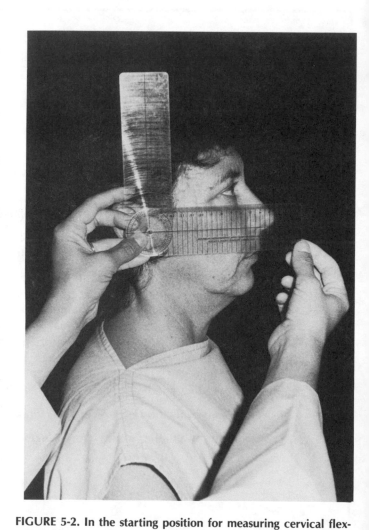

FIGURE 5-2. In the starting position for measuring cervical flexion, the examiner aligns the proximal goniometer arm so that it is perpendicular to the floor. The goniometer body is centered over the subject's external auditory meatus. The examiner aligns the distal arm with the base of the nares.

2. Align the proximal arm so that it is either perpendicular or parallel to the ground.
3. Align the distal arm with the base of the nares. If a tongue depressor is used, align the arm of the goniometer parallel to the longitudinal axis of the tongue depressor.

ALTERNATIVE MEASURING METHOD (Fig. 5-4)

A tape measure can be used to measure the distance between the tip of the chin and the sternal notch. Be sure that the subject's mouth remains closed.

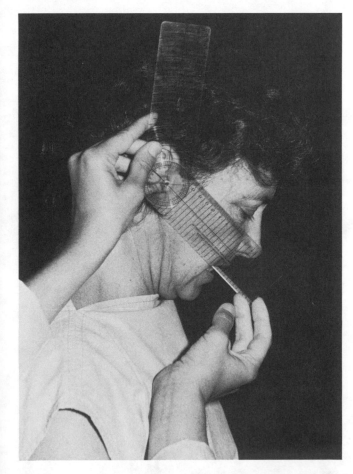

FIGURE 5-3. At the end of the ROM, the examiner's left hand aligns the proximal goniometer arm. The examiner uses her right hand to maintain alignment of the distal arm with the base of the nares. Also, the distal arm can be aligned parallel to the tongue depressor, which is being held between the subject's teeth.

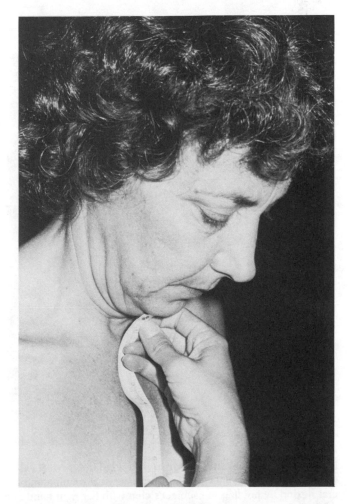

FIGURE 5-4. In the alternative method for measuring cervical flexion, the examiner uses a tape measure to determine the distance from the tip of the chin to the sternal notch.

EXTENSION

Motion occurs in the sagittal plane around a coronal axis.

RECOMMENDED TESTING POSITION, STABILIZATION, AND GONIOMETER ALIGNMENT
(Figs. 5-5, 5-6, and 5-7)

The testing position, stabilization, and alignment are the same as for measuring cervical flexion.

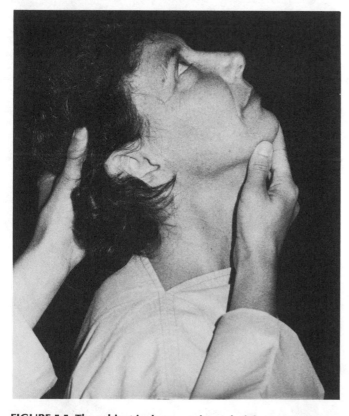

FIGURE 5-5. The subject is shown at the end of the cervical extension ROM. The examiner prevents both cervical rotation and lateral flexion by holding the subject's chin with her right hand and the subject's posterior head with her left hand. The back of the chair (which is not visible in the photograph) helps to prevent thoracic and lumbar extension.

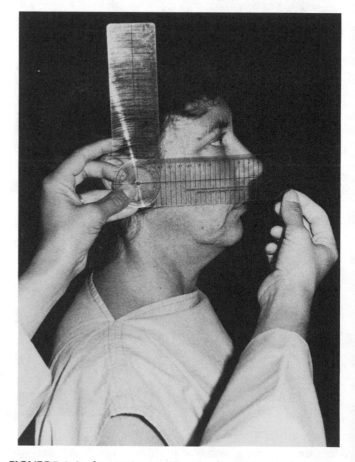

FIGURE 5-6. In the starting position for measuring cervical extension, goniometer alignment is the same as for measuring cervical flexion.

A tape measure can be used to measure the distance between the tip of the chin and the sternal notch. Be sure that the subject's mouth remains closed.

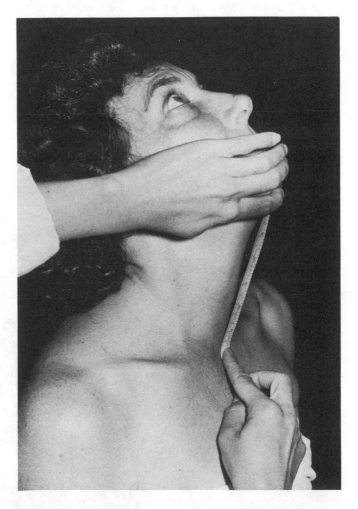

FIGURE 5-8. In the alternative method for measuring cervical extension, one end of the tape measure is placed on the tip of the subject's chin. The other end of the tape is placed at the subject's sternal notch. The distance between the two points of reference is recorded in inches or centimeters. The examiner measures the distance between the two reference points in the starting position prior to measuring the distance at the end of the ROM. The examiner records the beginning measurement as well as the measurement taken at the end of the ROM. The difference between these two measurements constitutes the ROM. Example: starting position: 2 inches; end ROM: 5 inches; ROM: 3 inches.

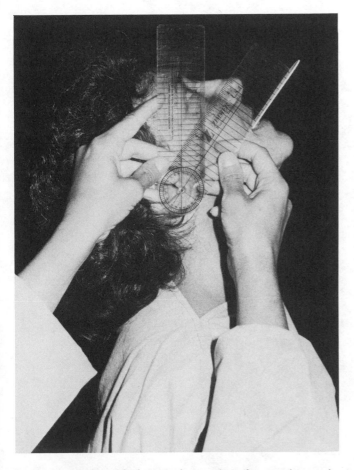

FIGURE 5-7. At the end of cervical extension, the examiner maintains the perpendicular alignment of the proximal goniometer arm with her left hand. The examiner's right hand aligns the distal arm with the base of the nares. A tongue depressor is being used to help align the distal arm.

LATERAL FLEXION

Motion occurs in the frontal plane around an anterior-posterior axis.

RECOMMENDED TESTING POSITION

Position the subject sitting, with the thoracic and lumbar spine well supported by the back of a chair. The cervical spine is positioned in 0 degrees of flexion, extension, and rotation.

STABILIZATION (Fig. 5-9)

Stabilize the shoulder girdle to prevent lateral flexion of the thoracic and lumbar spine.

GONIOMETER ALIGNMENT (Figs. 5-10 and 5-11)

1. Center the fulcrum of the goniometer over the spinous process of the C-7 vertebra.
2. Align the proximal arm with the spinous processes of the thoracic vertebrae so that the arm is perpendicular to the ground.
3. Align the distal arm with the dorsal midline of the head, using the occipital protuberance for reference.

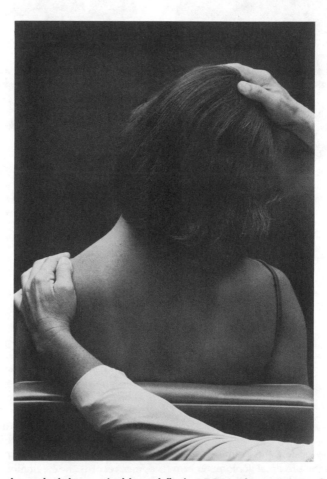

FIGURE 5-9. The subject is shown at the end of the cervical lateral flexion ROM. The examiner's left hand is holding the subject's left shoulder to prevent lateral flexion of the thoracic and lumbar spine. The examiner's right hand maintains cervical lateral flexion by pulling the subject's head laterally.

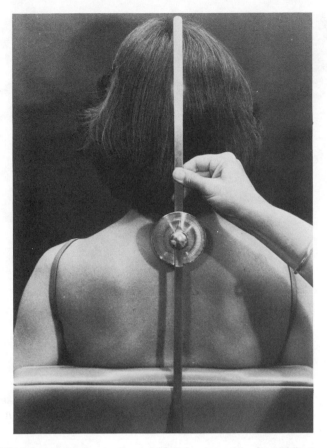

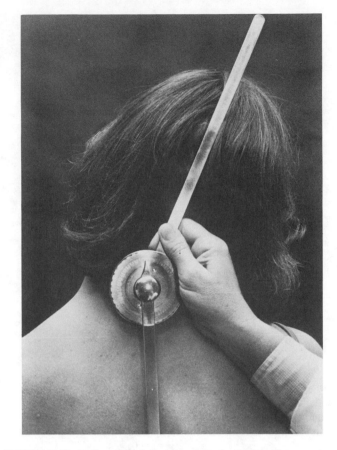

FIGURE 5-10. In the starting position for measuring lateral flexion, the examiner centers the body of the goniometer over the subject's seventh cervical vertebra. The freely movable proximal goniometer arm hangs so that it is perpendicular to the floor.

FIGURE 5-11. At the end of the lateral flexion ROM the examiner maintains alignment of the proximal goniometer arm with her right hand. Normally, the examiner would have one hand on the subject's head to maintain lateral flexion; however, in order to show the goniometer alignment in the photograph, the examiner is using only one hand.

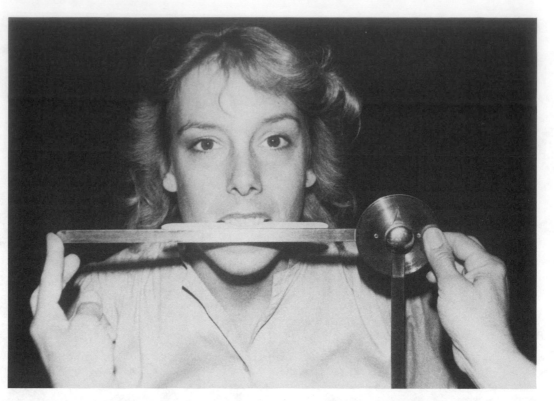

FIGURE 5-12. In the alternative method for measuring cervical lateral flexion, the subject is holding a tongue depressor between her teeth (the tongue depressor is almost completely hidden by the arm of the goniometer). The examiner aligns the distal goniometer arm parallel to the longitudinal axis of the tongue depressor. The proximal arm hangs so that it is perpendicular to the floor.

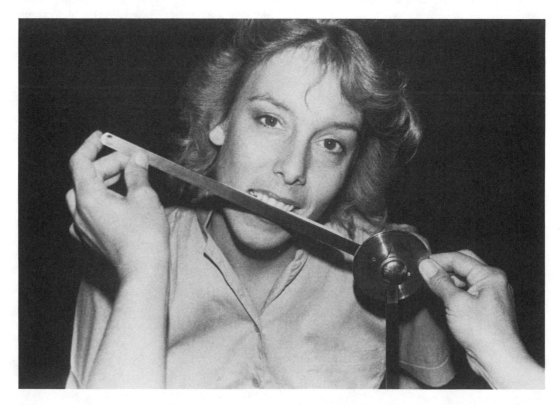

FIGURE 5-13. At the end of lateral flexion, the examiner maintains alignment of the distal goniometer arm with her left hand, while holding the fulcrum of the goniometer with her right hand.

ALTERNATIVE GONIOMETER ALIGNMENT
(Figs. 5-12 and 5-13)

A tongue depressor is held between the upper and lower teeth of both sides of the mouth.

1. Center the fulcrum of the goniometer near one end of the tongue depressor.
2. Align the proximal arm so that it is either perpendicular or parallel to the ground.
3. Align the distal arm with the longitudinal axis of the tongue depressor.

ALTERNATIVE MEASURING METHOD (Fig. 5-14)

A tape measure can be used to measure the distance between the mastoid process and the acromion process.

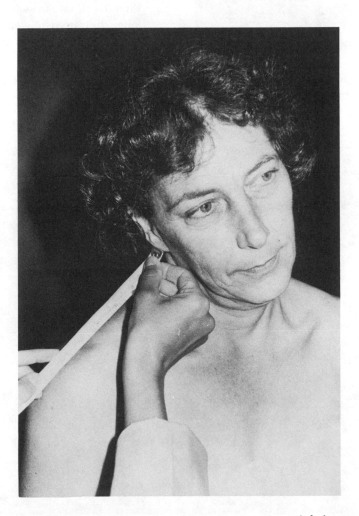

FIGURE 5-14. The distance between the subject's mastoid process and the acromion process is being used as a measure of cervical lateral flexion ROM. The examiner measures the distance between these two reference points both in the 0 starting position and at the end of the ROM. For recording of the measurements, follow the method described in Figure 5-8. In the above photograph, the subject is shown at the end of cervical lateral flexion ROM.

TESTING OF THE SPINE AND TEMPOROMANDIBULAR JOINT

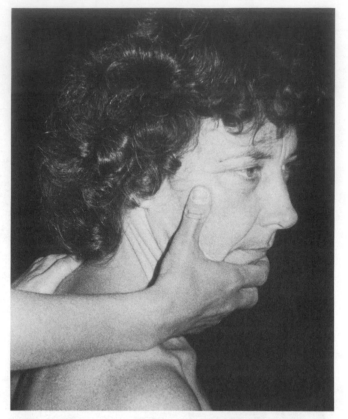

FIGURE 5-15. The subject is shown at the end of the cervical rotation ROM. The examiner's right hand maintains rotation and prevents cervical flexion and extension. The examiner's left hand is placed on the subject's left shoulder to prevent rotation of the thoracic and lumbar spine.

ROTATION

Motion occurs in the transverse plane around a vertical axis.

RECOMMENDED TESTING POSITION

Position the subject sitting, with the thoracic and lumbar spine well supported by the back of the chair. The cervical spine is positioned in 0 degrees of flexion, extension, and lateral flexion. A tongue depressor can be held between the front teeth for reference.

STABILIZATION (Fig. 5-15)

Stabilize the shoulder girdle to prevent rotation of the thoracic and lumbar spine.

GONIOMETER ALIGNMENT (Figs. 5-16 and 5-17)

1. Center the fulcrum of the goniometer over the center of the cranial aspect of the head.
2. Align the proximal arm parallel to an imaginary line between the two acromion processes.
3. Align the distal arm with the tip of the nose. If a tongue depressor is used, align the arm of the goniometer parallel to the longitudinal axis of the tongue depressor.

ALTERNATIVE MEASURING METHOD (Fig. 5-18)

A tape measure can be used to measure the distance between the tip of the chin and the acromion process.

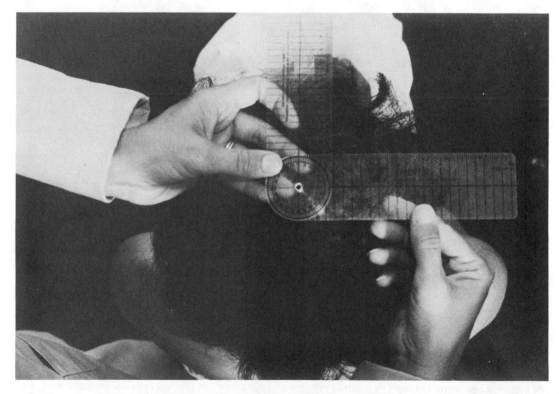

FIGURE 5-16. In order to accomplish initial goniometer alignment, the subject is seated in a low chair and the examiner stands in back of the subject. The examiner centers the fulcrum of the goniometer on top of the subject's head. The proximal goniometer arm is aligned parallel to an imaginary line between the subject's acromion processes. The examiner uses her left hand to align the distal goniometer arm with either the tip of the subject's nose or the tip of the tongue depressor.

MEASUREMENT OF JOINT MOTION: A GUIDE TO GONIOMETRY

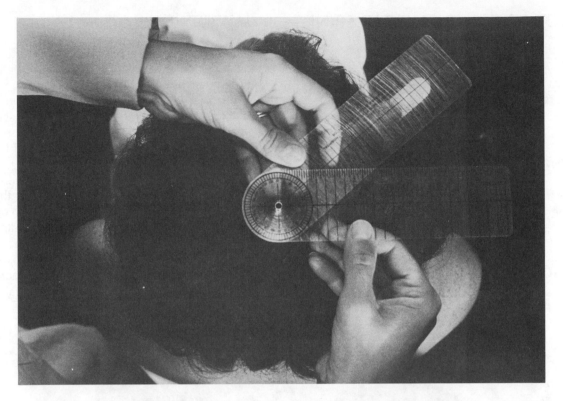

FIGURE 5-17. At the end of the range of right cervical rotation, the examiner's left hand maintains alignment of the distal goniometer arm with the tip of the subject's nose and with the tip of the tongue depressor. The examiner's right hand keeps the proximal arm aligned parallel to the subject's acromion processes.

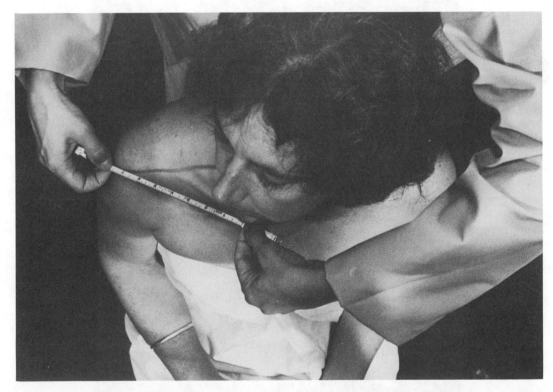

FIGURE 5-18. The subject is shown at the end of the right cervical rotation ROM. The examiner is using a tape measure to determine the distance between the tip of the subject's chin and the subject's right acromion process. The difference between measurements taken in the starting position and measurements taken at the end of the ROM provides the examiner with complete information about the subject's cervical rotation ROM to the right.

TESTING OF THE SPINE AND TEMPOROMANDIBULAR JOINT

THE THORACIC AND LUMBAR SPINE

FLEXION

Motion occurs in the sagittal plane around a coronal axis.

RECOMMENDED TESTING POSITION

Position the subject standing with the cervical, thoracic, and lumbar spine in 0 degrees of lateral flexion and rotation.

STABILIZATION (Fig. 5-19)

Stabilize the pelvis to prevent anterior tilting.

MEASUREMENT (Figs. 5-20 and 5-21)

The best method for determining the range of thoracic and lumbar flexion is to measure the distance between the spinous processes of C-7 and S-1 with a tape measure. The initial measurement is made with the subject in the 0 starting position, and the final measurement is made at the end of the range of motion. The difference between these two measurements indicates the amount of thoracic and lumbar flexion that is present.

Another method used by some examiners assesses thoracic and lumbar flexion by measuring, at the end of the range of motion, the distance between the tip of the subject's middle finger and the floor. This fingertip-to-floor or forward bending test combines spinal flexion and hip flexion, making it difficult to isolate and measure spinal flexion. Therefore, this test is not recommended for measuring thoracic and lumbar flexion[8] but can be used to assess general body flexibility.[32-34]

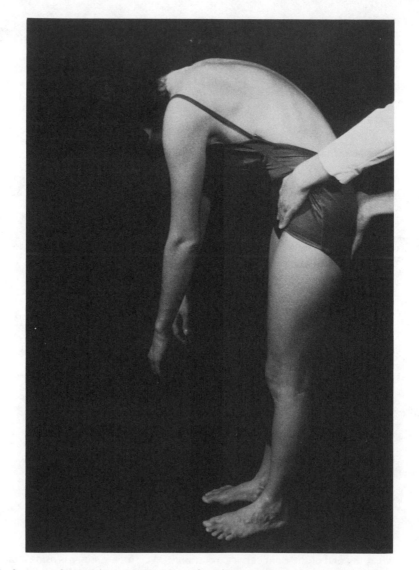

FIGURE 5-19. The subject is shown at the end of thoracic and lumbar flexion ROM. The examiner stabilizes the subject's pelvis to prevent anterior pelvic tilting while the subject bends forward.

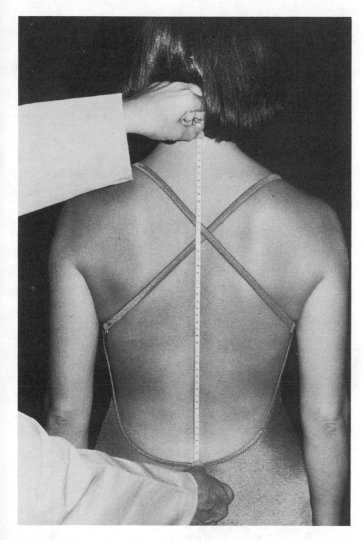

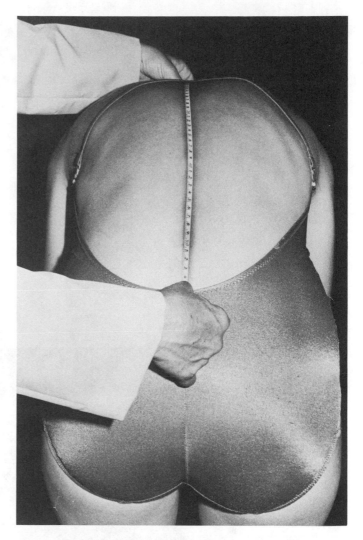

FIGURE 5-20. In the starting position for measuring thoracic and lumbar flexion, the examiner positions one end of the tape measure at the subject's seventh cervical vertebra. The examiner positions the other end of the tape measure over the first sacral vertebra.

FIGURE 5-21. At the end of the ROM, the examiner is maintaining the cervical end of the tape measure over the spinous process of the subject's seventh cervical vertebra. The sacral end of the tape measure is allowed to unwind to accommodate the spinal movement. The metal tape measure case is concealed in the examiner's right hand.

EXTENSION

Motion occurs in the sagittal plane around a coronal axis.

RECOMMENDED TESTING POSITION, STABILIZATION, AND MEASUREMENT (Figs. 5-22, 5-23, and 5-24)

The testing position, stabilization, and measurement are the same as for thoracic and lumbar flexion.

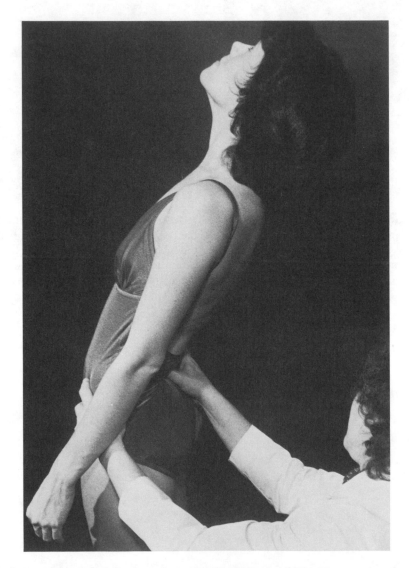

FIGURE 5-22. The subject is shown at the end of the thoracic and lumbar extension ROM. The examiner uses her left hand on the anterior pelvis and her right hand on the posterior pelvis to prevent posterior pelvic tilting. If the subject had balance problems or muscle weakness in her lower extremities, the measurements could be taken in either the prone or side-lying position.

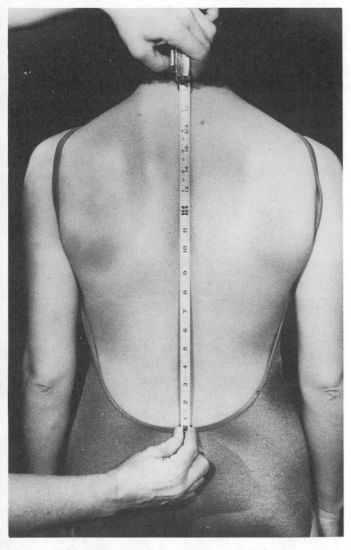 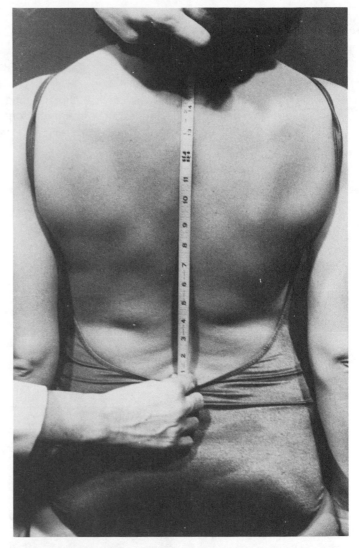

FIGURE 5-23. Positioning of the tape measure is the same as was used for measuring thoracic and lumbar flexion. In the photograph, the case of the tape measure is being held in the examiner's left hand. When the subject moves into extension, the tape slides into the casing.

FIGURE 5-24. At the end of thoracic and lumbar extension ROM the distance between the two reference points is less than it was in the starting position. The difference between the measurement taken in the starting position and the measurement taken at the end of the ROM constitutes the total ROM. The starting measurement, the end measurement, and the difference between these measurements are recorded in either inches or centimeters.

LATERAL FLEXION

Motion occurs in the frontal plane around an anterior-posterior axis.

RECOMMENDED TESTING POSITION

Position the subject standing, with the cervical, thoracic, and lumbar spine in 0 degrees of flexion, extension, and rotation.

STABILIZATION (Fig. 5-25)

Stabilize the pelvis to prevent lateral tilting.

GONIOMETER ALIGNMENT (Figs. 5-26 and 5-27)

1. Center the fulcrum of the goniometer over the posterior aspect of the spinous process of S-1.

2. Align the proximal arm so that it is perpendicular to the ground.

3. Align the distal arm with the posterior aspect of the spinous process of C-7.

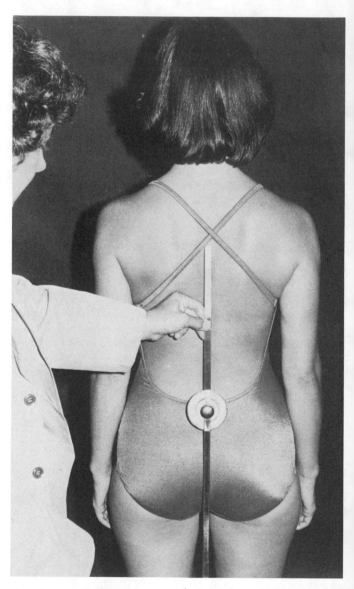

FIGURE 5-26. In the starting position for measuring thoracic and lumbar lateral flexion, the examiner centers the fulcrum of the goniometer over the spinous process of the subject's first sacral vertebra. The freely movable proximal goniometer arm hangs so that it is perpendicular to the floor. The examiner aligns the distal goniometer arm with the spinous process of the subject's seventh cervical vertebra.

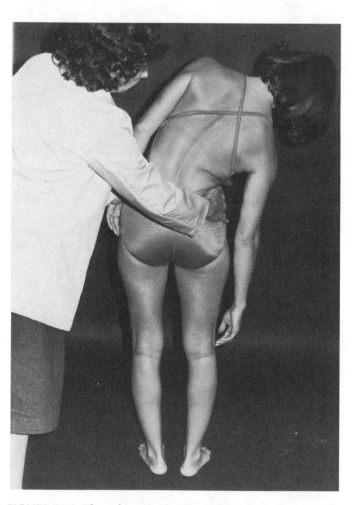

FIGURE 5-25. The subject is shown at the end of thoracic and lumbar lateral flexion ROM. The examiner places both hands on the subject's pelvis to prevent lateral pelvic tilting.

MEASUREMENT OF JOINT MOTION: A GUIDE TO GONIOMETRY

To measure the distance between the tip of the middle finger and the floor, both feet must be flat on the ground and the knees extended.

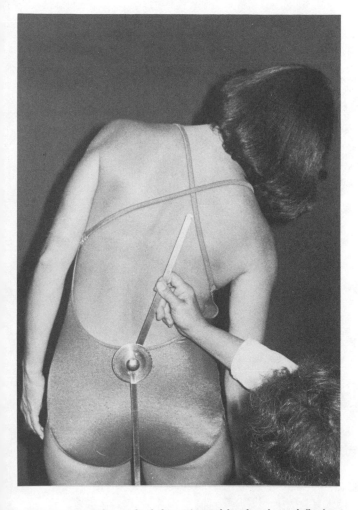

FIGURE 5-27. At the end of thoracic and lumbar lateral flexion, the examiner keeps the distal goniometer arm aligned with the subject's seventh cervical vertebra. The examiner makes no attempt to align the distal arm with the subject's vertebral column. As can be seen in the photograph, the lower thoracic and upper lumbar spine become convex to the left during right lateral flexion.

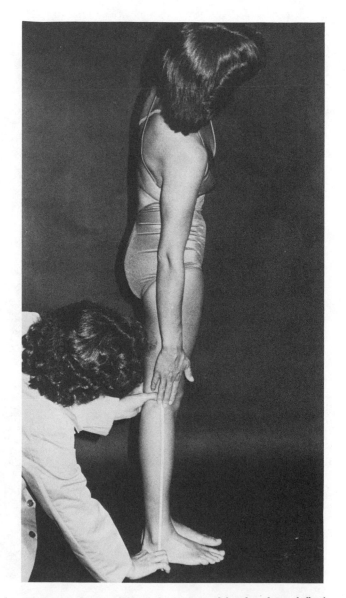

FIGURE 5-28. At the end of thoracic and lumbar lateral flexion ROM, the examiner is using a tape measure to determine the distance from the tip of the subject's third finger to the floor.

ROTATION

Motion occurs in the transverse plane around a vertical axis.

RECOMMENDED TESTING POSITION

Position the subject sitting, with the feet on the floor to help stabilize the pelvis. A seat without a back support is preferred so that rotation of the spine can occur freely. The cervical, thoracic, and lumbar spine are in 0 degrees of flexion, extension, and lateral flexion.

STABILIZATION (Fig. 5-29)

Stabilize the pelvis to prevent rotation. Avoid flexion, extension, and lateral flexion of the spine.

GONIOMETER ALIGNMENT (Figs. 5-30 and 5-31)

1. Center the fulcrum of the goniometer over the center of the cranial aspect of the head.
2. Align the proximal arm parallel to an imaginary line between the two prominent tubercles on the iliac crests.[10]
3. Align the distal arm with an imaginary line between the two acromion processes.

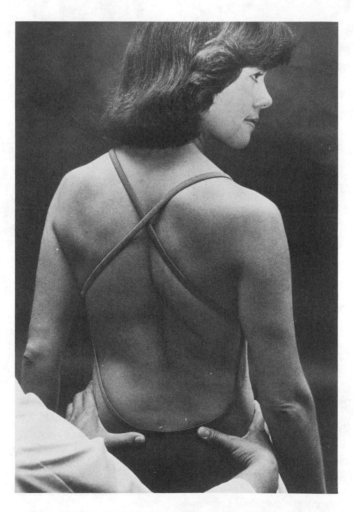

FIGURE 5-29. The subject is shown at the end of the thoracic and lumbar rotation ROM. The subject is seated on a low stool without a back rest so that spinal movement can occur without interference. The examiner positions her hands on the subject's iliac crests to prevent pelvic rotation.

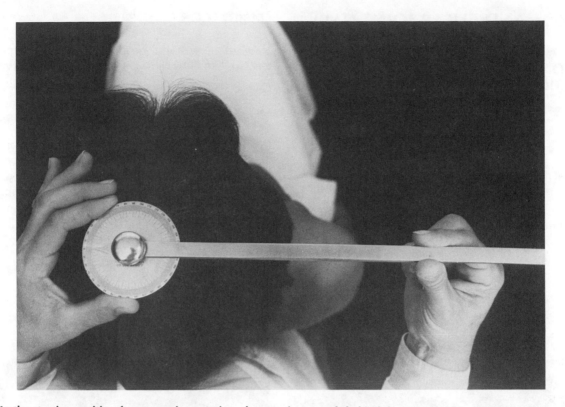

FIGURE 5-30. In the starting position for measuring rotation, the examiner stands behind the seated subject. The examiner positions the fulcrum of the goniometer on the superior aspect of the subject's head. The examiner's right hand is holding both arms of the goniometer aligned with the subject's acromion processes. The subject should be positioned so that the acromion processes are aligned directly over the iliac tubercles.

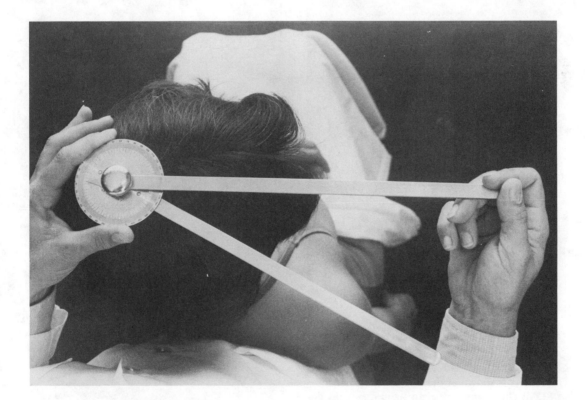

FIGURE 5-31. At the end of rotation, the examiner's right hand keeps the proximal goniometer arm aligned with the subject's iliac tubercles. The examiner aligns the distal goniometer arm with the subject's right acromion process.

TEMPOROMANDIBULAR JOINT (TMJ)

DEPRESSION OF THE LOWER JAW
(Opening Mouth)

Motion occurs in sagittal plane around a coronal axis.

RECOMMENDED TESTING POSITION

Position the subject sitting, with the cervical spine in 0 degrees of flexion, extension, lateral flexion, and rotation.

STABILIZATION (Fig. 5-32)

Stabilize the posterior head and neck to prevent flexion, extension, lateral flexion, and rotation of the cervical spine.

MEASUREMENT (Fig. 5-33)

Measure the distance between the upper central incisor teeth and the lower central incisor teeth with a tape measure or ruler. Normally, the lower jaw is reported to depress approximately 35 to 40 cm so that the subject's three fingers[10] or two knuckles[35] can be placed between the upper and lower central incisor teeth.

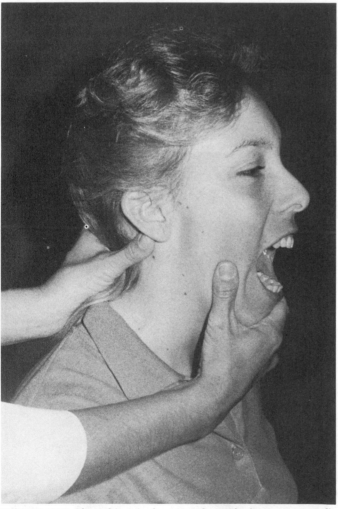

FIGURE 5-32. The subject is shown at the end of temporomandibular depression ROM. The examiner's right hand maintains depression by pulling the lower jaw inferiorly. The examiner's left hand holds the back of the subject's head to prevent cervical motion.

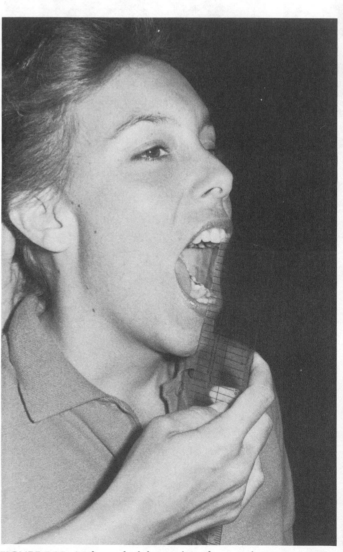

FIGURE 5-33. At the end of depression, the examiner uses an arm of a plastic goniometer to measure the distance between the subject's upper and lower central incisors.

ANTERIOR PROTRUSION OF THE LOWER JAW

Translatory motion occurs in the transverse plane.

RECOMMENDED TESTING POSITION

Position the subject sitting with the cervical spine in 0 degrees of flexion, extension, lateral flexion, and rotation. The TMJ is opened slightly.

STABILIZATION (Fig. 5-34)

Stabilize the posterior head and neck to prevent flexion, extension, lateral flexion, and rotation of the cervical spine.

MEASUREMENT (Fig. 5-35)

Measure the distance between the lower central incisor teeth and the upper central incisor teeth with a tape measure or ruler. Normally, the lower central incisor teeth are able to protrude beyond the upper central incisor teeth.[10,35]

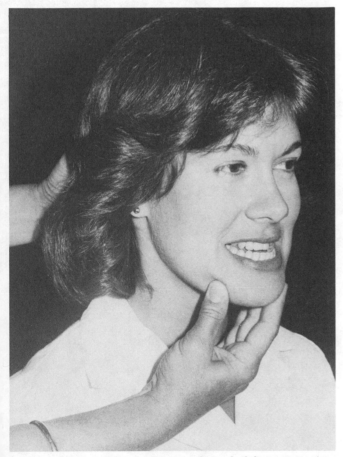

FIGURE 5-34. The subject is shown at the end of the temporomandibular anterior protrusion ROM. The examiner's left hand stabilizes the posterior aspect of the subject's head to prevent cervical motion. The examiner uses her right hand to maintain anterior protrusion.

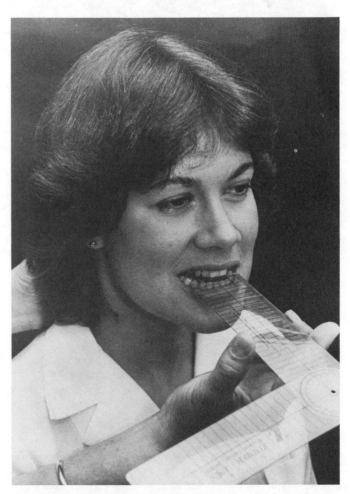

FIGURE 5-35. The examiner uses the end of a plastic goniometer to measure the distance between the subject's upper and lower central incisors. The subject maintains the motion.

LATERAL PROTRUSION OF THE LOWER JAW

Translatory motion occurs in the transverse plane.

RECOMMENDED TESTING POSITION AND STABILIZATION (Fig. 5-36)

The testing position and stabilization are the same as for anterior protrusion of the lower jaw.

MEASUREMENT (Fig. 5-37)

Measure the distance between the most lateral points of the lower and upper cuspid teeth or first bicuspid teeth with a tape measure or ruler. The amount of lateral movement to the right and left sides should be similar.[35]

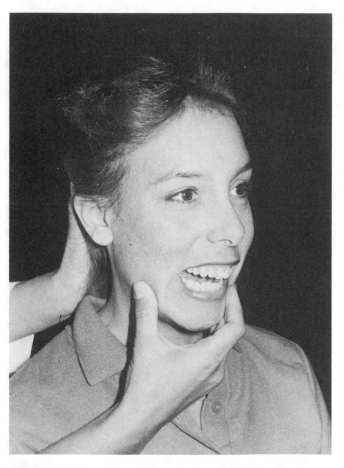

FIGURE 5-36. The subject is shown at the end of the temporomandibular lateral protrusion ROM. The examiner's left hand is placed on the back of the subject's head to prevent cervical motion. The examiner's right hand pulls the subject's lower jaw laterally to maintain lateral protrusion. The examiner avoids pulling the lower jaw into depression.

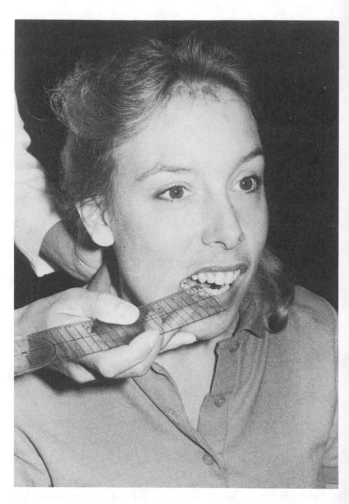

FIGURE 5-37. The examiner uses the end of a plastic goniometer to measure the distance between the upper and lower cuspids. The examiner maintains her grasp on the subject's head during the measurement.

REFERENCES

1. MOORE, ML: *Clinical assessment of joint motion.* In Licht, S: *Therapeutic Exercise.* Elizabeth Licht, New Haven, 1972.

2. BOONE, DC AND AZEN, SP: *Normal range of motion of joints in male subjects.* J Bone Joint Surg 61-A:756, 1979.

3. BOONE, DC, ET AL: *Reliability of goniometric measurements.* Phys Ther 58:1355, 1978.

4. BOONE, DC, WALKER, JM, AND PERRY, J: *Age and sex differences in lower extremity joint motion.* Paper presented at Annual Conference of American Physical Therapy Association, June 1981.

5. WOLF, SL, BASMAJIAN, JV, RUSSE, CT, ET AL: *Normative data on low back mobility and activity levels.* Am J Phys Med 58:217, 1979.

6. WAUGH, KL, MINKEL, JL, PARKER, R, ET AL: *Measuremernt of selected hip, knee, and ankle joint motions in newborns.* Phys Ther 63:1616, 1983.

7. FITZGERALD, GK, WYNYEEN, KJ, RHEAULT, W, ET AL: *Lumbar spinal range of motion.* Phys Ther 63:1776, 1983.

8. AMERICAN ACADEMY OF ORTHOPAEDIC SURGEONS: *Joint Motion: Method of Measuring and Recording.* American Academy of Orthopaedic Surgeons, Chicago, 1965.

9. KENDALL, HO AND MCCREARY, EK: *Muscles: Testing and Function,* ed 3. Williams & Wilkins, Baltimore, 1983.

10. HOPPENFELD, S: *Physical Examination of the Spine and Extremities.* Appleton-Century-Crofts, New York, 1976.

11. KAPANDJI, IA: *Physiology of the Joints,* Vol. 1, ed 2. Churchill-Livingstone, London, 1970.

12. KAPANDJI, IA: *Physiology of the Joints,* Vol. 2, ed 2. Williams & Wilkins, Baltimore, 1970.

13. KAPANDJI, IA: *Physiology of the Joints,* Vol. 3, ed 2. Churchill Livingstone, London, 1970.

14. ESCH, D AND LEPLEY, M: *Evaluation of Joint Motion: Method of Measurement and Recording.* University of Minnesota Press, Minneapolis, 1974.

15. TROMBLEY, CA AND SCOTT, AD: *Occupational Therapy for Physical Dysfunction.* Williams & Wilkins, Baltimore, 1977.

16. MCRAE, R: *Clinical-Orthopedic Examination.* Churchill Livingstone, New York.

17. CYRIAX, J: *Textbook of Orthopaedic Medicine: Diagnosis of Soft Tissue Lesions,* ed 6. Williams & Wilkins, Baltimore, 1975.

18. KALTENBORN, FM: *Mobilization of the Extremity Joints,* ed 3. Olaf Norlis Bokhandel, Oslo, 1982.

19. PARIS, SV: *Extremity Dysfunction and Mobilization.* Institute Press, Atlanta, 1980.

20. COOKSON, JC AND KENT, BE: *Orthopedic manual therapy—An overview.* Part I. Phys Ther 59:136, 1979.

21. GRAY, H AND GOSS, GM: *Gray's Anatomy of the Human Body.* Lea & Febiger, Philadelphia, 1982.

22. MOORE, KL: *Clinically Oriented Anatomy.* Williams & Wilkins, Baltimore, 1980.

23. STEINDLER, A: *Kinesiology of the Human Body.* Charles C Thomas, Springfield, Ill, 1955.

24. GOWITZKE, BA AND MILNER, M: *Understanding the Scientific Basis for Human Movement,* ed 2. Williams & Wilkins, Baltimore, 1980.

25. NORKIN, CC AND LEVANGIE, PK: *Joint Structure and Function.* FA Davis, Philadelphia, 1983.

26. LOW, JL: *The reliability of joint measurement.* Physiotherapy 67:227, 1976.

27. ROTHSTEIN, JM, MILLER, PJ, AND ROETTGER, F: *Goniometric reliability in a clinical setting.* Phys Ther 63:1611, 1983.

28. SPILMAN, HW AND PINKSTON, D: *Relation of test positions to radial and ulnar deviation.* Phys Ther 49:837, 1969.

29. THOMAS, DH AND LONG, C: *An electrogoniometer for the finger: A kinesiologic tracking device.* Am J Med Elec April-June: 96, 1964.

30. KETTELKAMP, DB, JOHNSON, RC, SMIDT, GL, ET AL: *An electrogoniometric study of knee motion in normal gait.* J Bone Joint Surg 52-A:775, 1970

31. TATA, JA, ET AL: *A variable axis electrogoniometer for measurement of single plane movement.* J Biomech 11:421, 1978.

32. KRAUS, H AND HIRSCHLAND, RP: *Minimum muscular fitness tests in school children.* Res Quart 25:178, 1954.

33. NICHOLAS, JA: *Risk factors, sports medicine and the orthopedic system: An overview.* J Sports Med 3:243, 1975

34. BRODIE, DA, BIRD, HA, AND WRIGHT, V: *Joint laxity in selected athletic populations.* Med Sci Sports Exercise 14:190, 1982.

35. FRIEDMAN, MH AND WEISBERG, J: *Application of orthopedic principles in evaluation of the temporomandibular joint.* Phys Ther 62:597, 1982.

APPENDICES

A. AVERAGE RANGES OF MOTION
B. JOINT MEASUREMENTS BY BODY POSITION

APPENDIX A

Average Ranges of Motion For the Upper Extremities

Joint	Motion	Amer Acad Ortho Surg[8]	Kendall McCreary[9]	Hoppenfeld[10]	Kapandji[11]
Shoulder					
	Flexion	0–180°	0–180°	0–90°	0–180°
	Extension	0–60	0–45	0–45	0–50
	Abduction	0–180	0–180	0–180	0–180
	Medial rotation	0–70	0–70	0–55	0–95
	Lateral rotation	0–90	0–90	0–45	0–80
Elbow	Flexion	0–150	0–145	0–150	0–145
Forearm					
	Pronation	0–80	0–90	0–90	0–85
	Supination	0–80	0–90	0–90	0–90
Wrist					
	Extension	0–70	0–70	0–70	0–85
	Flexion	0–80	0–80	0–80	0–85
	Radial Deviation	0–20	0–20	0–20	0–15
	Ulnar Deviation	0–30	0–35	0–30	
Thumb CMC					
	Abduction	0–70	0–80	0–70	0–50
	Flexion	0–15	0–45		
	Extension	0–20	0		
	Opposition	Tip of thumb to base or tip of fifth digit	Pad of thumb to pad of fifth digit	Tip of thumb to tip of fingers	
MCP					
	Flexion	0–50	0–60	0–50	0–80
IP					
	Flexion	0–80	0–80	0–90	0–80
Digit 2–5 MCP					
	Flexion	0–90	0–90		
	Extension	0–45		0–90	
	Abduction			0–45	
PIP	Flexion			0–20	
DIP	Flexion			0–100	
	Extension			0–90	
				0–10	

APPENDIX A—*continued*

Average Ranges of Motion For The Lower Extremities

Joint	Motion	Amer Acad Ortho Surg[8]	Kendall and McCreary[9]	Hoppenfeld[10]	Kapandji[12]
Hip					
	Flexion	0–120	0–125	0–135	0–120
	Extension	0–30	0–10	0–30	0–30
	Aduction	0–45	0–45	0–50	0–30
	Adduction	0–30	0–10	0–30	0–30
	Lat. Rot.	0–45	0–45	0–45	0–60
	Med. Rot.	0–45	0–45	0–35	0–30
Knee					
	Flexion	0–135	0–140	0–135	0–160
Ankle					
	Dorsiflex.	0–20	0–20	0–20	0–30
	Plantarflex.	0–50	0–45	0–50	0–50
	Inversion	0–35	0–35	– – – –	0–52
	Eversion	0–15	0–20	– – – –	0–30
Subtalar					
	Inversion	0–5		0–5	
	Eversion	0–5		0–5	
Transverse tarsal					
	Inversion	0–20		0–20	
	Eversion	0–10		0–10	
Toes					
First MTP					
	Flexion	0–45		0–45	0–50
	Extension	0–70		0–90	0–90
First IP					
	Flexion	0–90			
2–5 MTP					
	Flexion	0–40			0–50
	Extension	0–40			0–90
PIP	Flexion	0–35			
DIP	Flexion	0–30			
	Extension	0–60			

APPENDIX A—*continued*

Average Ranges of Motion For The Spine and Temporomandibular Joint

Joint	Motion	Amer Acad Ortho Surg[8]	Kendall and McCreary[9]	Hoppenfeld[10]	Kapandji[13]
Spine cervical					
	Flexion	0–45	0–45	Chin touches chest	0–40
	Extension	0–45	0–45	Look at ceiling	0–75
	Lat. Flexion	0–45		0–45	0–45
	Rotation	0–60		Chin in line with shoulder	0–50
Thoracic and Lumbar					
	Flexion	0–80 4 inches			0–105
	Extension	0–25			0–60
	Lat. Flexion	0–35			0–40
	Rotation	0–45			0–20
Temporomandibular					
	Depression			Three finger widths	
	Ant. Protrusion			Beyond lower teeth	
	Lat. Protrusion				

APPENDIX B

Joint Measurements by Body Position

	PRONE	SUPINE	SITTING	STANDING
SHOULDER	Extension	Flexion Abduction Medial Rotation Lateral Rotation	(Abduction)	
ELBOW		Flexion		
FOREARM			Pronation Supination	
WRIST			Flexion Extension Radial Deviation Ulnar Deviation	
HAND			All Motions	
HIP	Extension	Flexion Abduction Adduction	Medial Rotation Lateral Rotation	
KNEE	Flexion			
ANKLE/FOOT	Subtalar Inversion Subtalar Eversion	Dorsiflexion Plantarflexion Inversion Eversion Midtarsal Inversion Midtarsal Eversion	Dorsiflexion Plantarflexion Inversion Eversion Midtarsal Inversion Midtarsal Eversion	
TOES		All Motions	All Motions	
CERVICAL SPINE			Flexion Extension Lateral Flexion Rotation	Flexion Extension Lateral Flexion
THORACOLUMBAR SPINE			Rotation	

An italic page number indicates an illustration; a t after a page number indicates a table.

iliofemoral abduction and, 80, *81*
iliofemoral extension and, 78, *79*
iliofemoral flexion and, 76, *77*
iliofemoral lateral rotation and, 86, *87*
iliofemoral medial rotation and, 84, *85*
interphalangeal extension and, 74
interphalangeal flexion and, 72, *73*
lumbar spine lateral flexion and, 128, *129*
lumbar spine rotation and, 130, *131*
metacarpophalangeal abduction and, 54, *55*
metacarpophalangeal adduction and, 56
metacarpophalangeal extension and, 54, *55, 70, 71*
metacarpophalangeal flexion and, 52, *53, 70, 71*
metatarsophalangeal abduction and, 110
metatarsophalangeal adduction and, 110, *111*
metatarsophalangeal extension and, 108, *109*
metatarsophalangeal flexion and, 106, *107*
proximal interphalangeal extension and, 60
proximal interphalangeal flexion and, 58, *59*
radial deviation and, 48, *49*
subtalar eversion and, 100, *101*
subtalar inversion and, 98, *99*
tarsal eversion and, 96, *97*
tarsal inversion and, 94, *95*
thoracic spine lateral flexion and, 128, *129*
thoracic spine rotation and, 130, *131*
tibiofemoral extension and, 88, *89*
tibiofemoral flexion and, 88, *89*
transverse tarsal eversion and, 104, *105*
transverse tarsal inversion and, 102, *103*
ulnar deviation and, 50, *51*
wrist extension and, 46, *47*
wrist flexion and, 44, *45*
body of, 12, *13, 14*
full-circle, *14*
half-circle, *14*
materials used in, *13*
measurements with
recording of, 19, *20,* 21
parts of, 12, *13*
selection of, *15*
types of, 12, *13, 14*

HEAD, rotation of, *3*
Hindfoot
eversion of, 100
goniometer alignment for, 100, *101*
inversion of, 98
goniometer alignment for, 98, *99*
Hip(s)
abduction of, 80
goniometer alignment in, 80, *81*
adduction of, 82
goniometer alignment for, 82, *83*
extension of, 78
goniometer alignment for, 78, *79*
flexion of, 76
goniometer alignment for, 76, *77*
lateral rotation of, 86
goniometer alignment for, 86, *87*
medial rotation of, 84
goniometer alignment for, 84, *85*

INSTRUMENT(S)
measuring. *See* Goniometer(s).
Internal rotation. *See* Rotation, medial.
Inversion
of subtalar joint, 98, *98, 99*
of tarsal joints, 94, *94, 95*
of transverse tarsal joint, 102, *102, 103*

JAW(S)
lower
depression of, 132, *132*
protrusion of
anterior, 133, *133*
lateral, 134, *134*
Joint(s)
ankle. *See* Joint(s), talocrural; *and* Ankle(s).
carpometacarpal
abduction of, 66
goniometer alignment for, 66, *67*
adduction of, 66
extension of, 64
goniometer alignment for, 64, *65*
flexion of, 62
opposition of, 68
goniometer alignment for, 68, *69*
distal interphalangeal
extension of
goniometer alignment for, 61
flexion of
goniometer alignment for, 61
glenohumeral
abduction of
goniometer alignment for, 32–33, *32, 33*
adduction of, 33
extension of
goniometer alignment for, 28, *29*
flexion of, 26, *26, 27*
goniometer alignment for, 26, *27*
internal rotation of. *See* Joint(s), glenohumeral, medial rotation of.
lateral rotation of
goniometer alignment for, 36, *37*
medial rotation of
goniometer alignment for, 34, *35*
humeroradial
extension of, 38
goniometer alignment for, 38, *39*
flexion of, 38
goniometer alignment for, 38, *39*
humeroulnar
extension of, 38
goniometer alignment for, 38, *39*
flexion of, 38
goniometer alignment for, 38, *39*
iliofemoral
abduction of, 80
goniometer alignment for, 80, *81*
adduction of, 82
goniometer alignment for, 82, *83*
extension of, 78
goniometer alignment for, 78, *79*
flexion of, 76
goniometer alignment for, 76, *77*